D0049062

GINSENG,
the Divine Root

GINSENG,

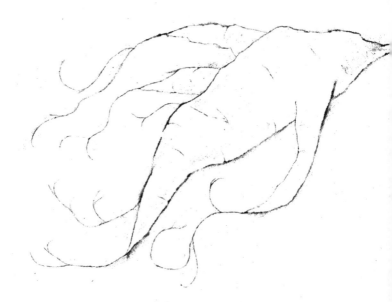

the Divine Root

DAVID A. TAYLOR

ALGONQUIN BOOKS OF CHAPEL HILL 2006

Published by

ALGONQUIN BOOKS OF CHAPEL HILL

Post Office Box 2225

Chapel Hill, North Carolina 27515-2225

a division of

Workman Publishing

708 Broadway

New York, New York 10003

Printed in the United States of America.

Published simultaneously in Canada by Thomas Allen & Son Limited.

Design by Anne Winslow.

Illustration on pp. ii–iii by Laura Williams.

Library of Congress Cataloging-in-Publication Data

Taylor, David A., 1961–

Ginseng, the divine root / David A. Taylor.—1st ed.

p. cm.

Includes bibliographical references and index.

ISBN-13: 978-1-56512-401-1; ISBN-10: 1-56512-401-4

1. Ginseng—Therapeutic use. 2. Ginseng. 3. Herbs—Therapeutic use. I. Title.

RS165.G45T39 2006

615'.32384—dc22   2005052726

10 9 8 7 6 5 4 3 2 1

First Edition

For my parents,
Bill and Nancy Taylor

SEN. ROCKEFELLER: "... I would say to the good senator from New York, if you're looking for good ginseng, come to West Virginia, sir. We have the best."

SEN. MOYNIHAN: "There are arguments. Delaware County, New York, is—(laughter)—still ahead among the Chinese elite, no doubt about it. Chairman Mao smoked only ginseng cigarettes from Delaware County. West Virginia is close. (Laughter.)"

—Capitol Hill hearing, June 6, 1996

✺

"Hell, I wasn't aiming on shooting nothing today, I's just looking for sang," he said. "Got me a alimony payment due."

"Oh, well, then," she said, nodding seriously, "good thing you brought that rifle. Sang plants can get real mean in breeding season."

—BARBARA KINGSOLVER, *Prodigal Summer,* 2000

✺

"Do you think I wanted to walk with this woman? She was talking about ginseng for an hour and a half!"

—LARRY DAVID, *Curb Your Enthusiasm,* 1999

Contents

GINSENG,
the Divine Root

INTRODUCTION

The Cherokees speak of the plant as a sentient being . . .
able to make itself invisible to those unworthy to gather it.
—WILLIAM BARTRAM, naturalist, Philadelphia, 1791

RESTING ON MY DESK is a single dried ginseng root. It looks small and insubstantial, a shriveled, pale brown finger against a dark background. This one is four years old and came from a craft shop in Cherokee, North Carolina.

Few Americans would recognize this root as ginseng. Most people think of ginseng as a Chinese herb used in energy-boosting food supplements. A visit to a health-food super-market reveals a staggering array of them. The soft-drink aisle launches a rainbow brigade of shrink-wrapped bottles that list ginseng on their labels. The tea section has its own universe of ginseng items, from Yogi Tea to American Ginzing herbal tea. Even industry stalwart Lipton sells yellow boxes of Lemon Gin-seng tea bags. In the dietary supplement section, shelves and shelves are devoted to ginseng capsules and tinctures of all kinds, often packaged with images of white-haired Asian philosophers or powerful dragons.

The root on my desk, however, is simply American ginseng, *Panax quinquefolius,* a native to North American forests and vir-tually identical to its sister in Asia, *Panax ginseng.* Asian ginseng has indeed been used for several thousand years as a popular health tonic. Less known is the fact that for nearly three centuries, this surprising family resemblance between the two plants has led American ginseng to navigate a labyrinthine passage around the world.

This ginseng root holds other surprises. For one thing, it's harder than you'd expect of an herb. Biting off a piece is like snapping a half-inch wooden dowel in two. Even before a small piece reaches my mouth, I smell the soil it came from. I place the root on my tongue and the tannic tang reminds me vaguely of cloves. Not exactly a pleasant taste, it's been described as slightly aromatic, or like licorice root. The flavor evokes an earlier age, a time of sarsaparilla and anise seed. The root catches on my teeth, and within a minute its woody texture gives way to fibrous threads.

IF YOU LIVE NEAR mountains in the eastern half of North America, you can wander the woods for days, hoping to find a ginseng plant in the wild. I have kept my eyes open on many hikes where the terrain looked right: shady, north-facing slopes, mossy rock outcroppings, clusters of hardwood trees. But ginseng is a shy creature. Novice visitors always need an introduction from someone who knows the herb well. It's not like other famous forest residents. Oak and walnut trees are easily recognizable, lording over the forest like statuesque movie stars. Ginseng isn't like that. It blends in easily with other plants, such as poison oak. Yet a Park Service botanist who has tromped the Great Smokies for years says that of all the rare plants in the woods—of all the ones that she could choose in the forest's vastness—ginseng is her favorite. She enjoys tracking its aboveground life as it races through the seasons, from a single stem in spring, to a flush of leaves, to sports-car-red berries that last just a week in mid-summer. By fall, its leaves turn a pale yellow before the plant seems to disappear altogether.

Below the soil, however, the root (technically, a rhizome) continues to develop with painfully slow deliberation. Each year adds a wrinkle on its neck, establishing a unique signature, like a tree's rings. And while that signature might seem meaningless hidden in the forest, it will gain significance later. For generations of collectors who call themselves ginsengers, that root and its wild signatures have been an excellent reason for an autumn walk in the woods. People in Pocahontas County, West Virginia, can still point to farms that were bought with ginseng money. More often, digging ginseng roots and selling them to a buyer in a bait shop down the road produced enough cash to buy Christmas gifts or school supplies. When the crunch of dead leaves and sunlight against bare tree trunks signaled darker days coming, ginseng promised that Christmas bonus.

American ginsengers through the centuries were happy to collect the roots to sell, but it was rare for them to chew the root themselves. And there's still a good deal of debate among American doctors about whether ginseng does any good. Depending on who you ask, ginseng either works to catalyze the body's vital energy, or it acts as a mild tonic and antioxidant, or it's a fraud. Some U.S. researchers have found that certain chemicals in American ginseng may protect brain cells against degenerative conditions like Parkinson's disease. No one denies, though, that ginseng has, at least, a very powerful effect on the imagination. Few elements of nature have inspired such an enormous range of creative responses as ginseng. This refers not only to farmers who have tried to grow it and researchers who have devised new ways to study the herb's chemical compounds, but also to the hucksters who for so long hawked ginseng as an aphrodisiac. (The world of ginseng holds an abundance of lowbrow imagination. Seedy massage parlor owners in Hong Kong's Kowloon Tong have figured out how to infuse ginseng into their sauna baths to boost revenues, and the ways to invoke ginseng in fraudulent mail-order schemes that promise better sexual performance are seemingly infinite.) Ginseng has inspired poems, stories, novels by Jack London and others, dance numbers, paintings, and the slide-guitar sounds of "Ginseng Sullivan," a song that recounts the trials of a soul digging ginseng in cold, hard ground.

Few plants have been as vividly anthropomorphized as the one known in Chinese as the "divine herb," the "king of herbs," and the "returned cinnabar with the wrinkled face." Whether in an Appalachian ginsenger's tale or a Chinese legend, stories about ginseng testify to an amazement at the plant's capacity to endure, and they speak to our own aspirations for weathering change. Wild ginseng has grown scarce, and the ginsenger's way of life, passed from father to son, may be passing. But in many places people still talk of the plant as having a thrill to it.

"I love to fool with that ginseng," George Albright, a digger in West Virginia, told me. "You don't know what it's going to do."

Albright had led me up a slope into the woods behind his house. A freight train echoed in the morning air, a reminder that we were in coal country, but soon we were surrounded by Appalachian deciduous forest, bright green after weeks of rain. Albright had hunted ginseng in this part of West Virginia for over fifty years. As a boy, he spent most of his time in the woods, and now that he was retired, he had returned to them. He knew that pound for pound, wild ginseng was one of the most valuable commodities in those mountains, and that the plant's value had put it on the endangered species list. He talked about how the root was saved only by being so hard to find. Some of his neighbors speculate that Albright has an extra gland that helps him find it.

After we walked a distance under the forest canopy, he stopped and bent down low. "Here," he said. Suddenly we were peering down on a four-prong ginseng plant. Its slender stem rose about six inches above the ground and branched into four smaller ones, each with a cluster of five arrow-shaped leaves. Albright set about the careful operation of unearthing the root, gently scraping away the dirt. When he finally held it up, the six-inch-long root twisted in every direction, with odd and irregular bends. A ginseng dealer at the bait shop down the road might pay Albright a few dollars for it, but a customer in a shop in San Francisco or Hong Kong would pay at least ten times more for a wild root like that.

In fact, this was another creative response to ginseng. Strictly speaking, this slender prize wasn't wild ginseng. Yes, it was growing without fertilizers or crop rows in its native forest, but it had help: George had sown the seed himself. This was "simulated-wild" ginseng, an ingenious wrinkle in the market that could pay off for ginsengers and breathe new life into American forests. George had made a domesticated plant look wild, and got a better price for it. Since boyhood, ginseng had given him a way to look at his forest with a sense of magic and purpose. Now he re-paid it with a creative approach that made it more abundant.

Not far from George Albright's land, Daniel Boone had dug ginseng in the 1780s and sold it to Philadelphia merchants with ships bound for China. Ever since that time, American ginseng has ridden waves of prosperity, crime, and human frailty. The ginseng trade fed the fortune of America's first millionaire, ensnared peasants in back-breaking work, promised long life to kings in Europe and Asia, and lured others to prison and even death.

Ginseng's expressive contortions invite the attention of millions. That shape! That aroma! The expectation of a quickened pulse, and the scent of the soil. Ginseng takes people to the limits of speech. How do you describe a taste precisely? How do you translate *vital energy*? "Ginseng's mystery defies logic and Western thinking," Bob Beyfuss, an agricultural agent, told me. "It satisfies a need that cannot be defined, much like sex." There have been houses that have burned down where the most-grieved loss was an old ginseng root in a glass case. "I can remember a whole lot of times digging 'sang," one ginsenger told me, "but I can't remember much else from when I was little."

DURING FOUR YEARS I spent in Asia as a science editor, I never suspected such an eventful past or intense connection between that part of the world and my home state of Virginia. Ginseng has something of a forgotten history, which began when Jesuit missionaries made the discovery that American ginseng was nearly identical to the Asian ginseng so treasured in China. Through the eighteenth and nineteenth centuries, the plant held an honored place in American life, commerce, foreign relations, and medicine, and reflected attitudes that can be hard for many today to fathom. Ginseng hunting, often a bond between father and son, remained a vital part of rural livelihoods well into the 1900s. Its abundance and value helped thousands of poor families make a living, people whom *The New York Times* derided as "shiftless, roving people, wholly incapable of keeping up with the march of modern progress."

This hidden history is one of thousands among medicines used by people around the globe. When they get sick, most of the world's population still turns to plants, not packaged pharmaceuticals. Ethnobotanists say that plants gain value as medicine only after many generations of people using them for food and other needs. Throughout the Americas and Africa, in Europe and Asia, medicinal plants have left deep memories of tastes and sensations. These plants are collected mostly from the wild and move through the world on informal pathways, unchecked by customs agents or health regulations. Ginseng, like many others, faces the possibility that it will not survive in the wild for much longer. If it doesn't, strands of our own history will be lost.

Meanwhile, every fall, American ginseng continues to get shepherded along routes that lead from forests to the world's cities and suburbs, passing through an eclectic assortment of hands. Some roots wind up in court as evidence, some in the clinics of Cedars-Sinai Hospital in Los Angeles. American ginseng roots, both wild and farm-grown, are shipped to South America, Europe, and Asia. In Hong Kong, a street crammed with traditional medicine shops sells wooden bins full of the root, while high above on the steep hillside in a shiny university lab, scientists track its chemical fingerprints. The history of this modest plant brings together Iroquois botanical knowledge and the theory of continental drift, diverse histories of Jesuit studies, ethnography and fur trapping, acupuncture and old-time musicians, fraud and folklore. Perhaps no other plant encompasses quite this range and intensity of human experience.

This book is about a plant poised between the danger of the wild and the safety of domestication, and is a picaresque of what life is like for a species balancing between extinction and stardom.

Throughout one fall and winter, I followed American ginseng. From upstate New York, it led me down North America's eastern mountains to North Carolina, westward to the Mississippi River, and across the Pacific to Hong Kong and southern China. The plant, like a secret handshake or an epic told by a series of storytellers, introduced me to trappers in West Virginia, Harvard-trained medical researchers, Cherokee elders, gourmet chefs, smugglers, law-enforcement officers, cultural anthropologists and history professors, and a business mogul or two. I set out on ginseng's wild journey through the world, and discovered a path it has charted through human nature.

A Note on Terms

WILD GINSENG refers to the plant as it grows in its native forest, with no help from people. Wild ginseng commands the highest price, and is limited to the plant's native range. For American ginseng *(Panax quinquefolius)*, that basically means mountains east of the Mississippi River, although it does grow in patches as far west as Nebraska. Wild Asian ginseng *(Panax ginseng)* is found only in northeastern China, Korea, and parts of Siberia.

Other ginseng relatives are: *Panax notoginseng,* found in China as *san chi* or *tien chi* ginseng; *Panax japonicum,* or Japanese ginseng and found only in Japan; and *Panax trifolium,* known as dwarf ginseng. There is a less documented basis for these plants than for the main two ginseng species, and they are not nearly as valuable. *Eleutherococcus senticosus,* sometimes called Siberian ginseng, is not a true ginseng, but a relative in the same plant family; it has almost no ginsenosides (the active chemical compounds in *Panax* species), and labeling rules now prohibit it from being marketed under the name "ginseng."

CULTIVATED GINSENG is the farm-grown version, which requires shade arbors, chemical pesticides and fungicides, and intense labor. For generations it was primarily cultivated in Wisconsin, but it is now widely grown in China and on farms around the world.

SIMULATED-WILD GINSENG is a fairly new, middle category (although experts maintain that thousands of years ago, Koreans grew simulated-wild ginseng in forests, too). Promoted as an ecologically sustainable alternative to cultivated ginseng, simulated-wild plants grow from seed sown by people in forest conditions that mimic the habitat of wild ginseng. Simulated-wild ginseng is mainly limited to areas where ginseng also grows wild — in America, in forests east of the Mississippi — and it is raised with no or very few chemicals or tilling. Markets in Asia have been slow to acknowledge this as a separate category; simulated-wild roots are easily mistaken for wild roots and command a higher price than cultivated roots.

ONE

The Root at Hand

*Wisdom . . . requires patience, persistence, curiosity
and hard work. These are precisely the same requisites
for growing ginseng.*

—Bob Beyfuss, *American Ginseng Production in the 21st Century*

O<small>N A CRISP DAY</small> in September 2002, a few maples flared
red against the green ridge on the east bank of the Hudson River and signaled the start of ginseng season. On the west
bank, two festival tents flapped in a breeze at Catskill Point
park, in the village of Catskill, New York. Food vendors in the
Dutchman's Galley were doing brisk business in hot dogs and
schnitzel, and the festival was drawing an eclectic assortment of
people. The organizers had sent announcements to farms all
over the surrounding county and posted handbills in neighborhoods throughout New York City, two hours south. They translated the flyers into Chinese and Korean, invited New Age
medicine specialists and dairy farmers, and arranged for entertainment, from acoustic duos to gospel choirs. Now, as a man
in a kilt droned away on bagpipes in the center of the fairground, buses arrived in the parking lot, hauling scores of people from Manhattan's Chinatown.

What brought them all together was ginseng, a plant at home on two continents, treasured in one for millennia and traded in the other for centuries, and still something of an enigma even to those who know it best. This was Catskill's first annual Ginseng Festival, but the plant was no newcomer here.

Ginseng is so old that scientists call members of its genus "living fossils," meaning plants that have remained unchanged since the first appearance of angiosperms more than 65 million years ago. Ginseng's family, Araliaceae, is among the oldest known group of angiosperms. (Angiosperms are flowering plants with enclosed seeds, the group that dominates the plant world today: everything from poppies to apple trees.) Outlines of *Panax* plants have appeared etched in stones found in Colorado dating back at least to the Oligocene Epoch, which began 38 million years ago.

Geobotanists say ginseng goes back seventy million years, when the two *Panax* species began as one. (The name, like *panacea,* stems from the Greek word for "cure.") Back then, a megacontinent known as Laurasia dominated the Northern Hemisphere and was blanketed by a thick deciduous forest. That explains why over three quarters of the plant families native to China's eastern Hubei Province are also native to the Carolinas. Magnolias, whose scent I always associated with Faulkner and the American South, abound in East Asia—over fifty species. Hydrangeas, too.

North America split off from Laurasia about fifty million years ago, and the Pacific slowly widened. At the end of the Miocene Age, about two million years ago, the western half of North America buckled and a tumultuous climate shredded the plant habitats in the American West. Fragmented populations in that region dwindled below their survival threshold and died out, but in the more stable terrain east of the Mississippi, forests remained nearly intact and still resembled those of northeast Asia. Eventually, people on both sides of the new ocean started using the plants that grew near them. The Cherokee used *Jeffersonia diphylla,* a small herb found in forests from Ontario down to North Carolina, as a poultice for sores and inflammations, and the Iroquois boiled the plant to treat diarrhea. That plant's Asian relative, *Jeffersonia dubia,* became a folk cure for stomach problems in northern China and Korea. And people on both sides of the Pacific started using ginseng.

Asian ginseng and American ginseng adapted slightly differently to their respective homes, with subtle variations in chemistry. The two have been described as the "twin pillars of both traditional and modern herbal medicine: the Asian a stimulant, the American a relaxant; the Asian a virility booster, the American a feminine tonic; the Asian an embodiment of yang, the American of yin."

AT THE FESTIVAL, THE first tent was crowded with displays of ginseng products and memorabilia from different eras. A local couple was handing out Ziploc bags of maple-chip candy coated in ginseng syrup, so a teenaged girl asked for a taste. "Sweet!" she said. Then her smile turned into a sour face as the bitter aftertaste hit.

Two Korean businessmen at a nearby booth outlined their strategy for exporting American ginseng to Asia. They were also there to buy American ginseng roots at an incredibly high price, as it turned out. They paid several local diggers about $1,500 per pound for twenty-five-year-old wild ginseng roots. That was three times the peak price that most North American diggers would see that season.

A camera crew wearing baseball caps with the gold National Geographic logo was filming an interview with a young Korean-American couple who had driven three hours from Long Island. The camera operator zoomed in as the woman bit into a long, pale tendril of American ginseng. She smiled and said it tasted just like Korean ginseng, which has been cultivated there at least since the sixteenth century. She held it out for her husband to take a bite.

The second tent was so crowded that it resembled a huge white millipede, with human legs poking from under the back flap. Inside, a bearded man spoke above the noise of the bag-piper and the bucking tent flaps. He spoke in a quiet drawl to a mix of New Agers, farmers, and city people about the best soil medium for germinating ginseng seeds—aquarium sand—and told the rapt audience how to apply fungicidal sprays. Suddenly a man in the back row strode forward as if he was going to storm the stage. He had a shock of flowing white hair and a huge plant tattoo on his right bicep. A few people in the crowd would later recall that moment with some alarm. "He looked like this wild Jack Nicholson character," one said, "moving closer so he could heckle the speaker."

The wild man was Bob Beyfuss (rhymes with *typhus*), the res-ident ginseng expert and festival organizer, preparing to intro-duce the next presenters.

• • •

SEVERAL WEEKS BEFORE THE festival, I had visited Beyfuss in the Greene County office building west of Catskill for the first ginseng hunt of the season. Every surface in his office was covered, with papers but also with photos of his grown children, ginseng roots carved with faces, and books on ginseng—everything from its trade and medicinal use to an 1881 manual on its growth and diseases. The walls held mounted fish, a stuffed red-tail hawk perched behind the door, certificates (one announced that Beyfuss was an "Official Fun Person"), and a small gold marker warning THIS ANIMAL IS DANGEROUS.

The tattoo on his arm, he said, was a midlife crisis: a full-color, life-size illustration of a huge five-prong ginseng plant, from leaves to root. Ginseng diggers everywhere talk about prongs—the bracts that branch off from the main stem and give a rough idea of the plant's age. One-prongs are a year old, two-prongs are two years, and a four-prong generally signals a plant four years old or older. After four years, a plant rarely adds prongs, so to tell the age you have to dig up the root and count the scars that gather on its neck, one every year. Beyfuss had a botanical illustrator paint the image from one of his own plants, a nine-year-old. Then a tattoo artist needed most of a day to transfer the illustration to Beyfuss's arm. Beyfuss hiked up his blue shirt sleeve to reveal the botanically correct image: a flush of leaves on his shoulder in rich greens, the red berries full, and the brown, branchy root only slightly smaller than it should have been.

Beyfuss had been involved with ginseng for twenty years, starting at a low point in his life. In 1984 he had been working as a county agricultural agent for seven years and his marriage had just ended. He was going back to school for a master's degree after a long hiatus, and he felt old among the other graduate students. Plus, the atmosphere at Cornell was much more competitive and stressful than at Rutgers, where he had gotten his undergraduate degree. He was commuting two hours each way from his day job in Greene County. With the added strain of studying, he was a wreck.

He started taking ginseng, chewing a bit of root daily, and found that despite getting less sleep, he could keep going through a full schedule of work, study, and almost-daily racquetball games. Ginseng seemed to cut his stress load, improve his energy, and, he thought, help him to lose weight.

Ginseng also gave him a niche at Cornell, where the agriculture program is world famous and the precedents were daunting. After months of searching for a thesis topic, Beyfuss found that most natural products and ecosystems already had their champions there. "At Cornell, they know everything about everything," he told me. "Nobody knew *nothing* about ginseng."

That itself was strange, since just a century before, upstate New York had been home to the first popular efforts to cultivate ginseng outside its native forests, on farmland. But Beyfuss found that knowledge of ginseng has historically gone through cycles of fascination and complete indifference. At the start of the twentieth century, growing ginseng for the China market was a hot focus of scientific research and the subject of several USDA manuals. By mid-century it was all but forgotten. Interest in digging the wild root would spike in one locality for a while, then die down until just a handful of people even remembered what ginseng looked like. These cycles are not unique to ginseng, but like so much else about the plant, they seem more pronounced.

For professional foresters, ginseng has always fallen into a category awkwardly labeled *nontimber forest products,* which covers everything from mushrooms to maple syrup, rubber to log moss, and wildflowers to wild turkeys. Modern forestry has a primary focus on timber; everything else is secondary. Yet history is full of instances where people considered other forest items more essential than wood. Gum arabic, a resin from the acacia tree in the Sudan, was a major commodity in ancient Egypt for its use in paints and the mummifying process. Olive oil and cork, from the bark of the cork tree, drove trade in the Mediterranean. In 300 BC wild silphion was so recognizable and valuable as medicine and commodity in Cyrene (present-day Libya) that coins were embossed with the plant's image. Forest plants often accrued cultural meaning and importance, too.

Beyfuss wrote his thesis on ginseng's history, medicinal uses, and cultivation. He described how to prepare the seeds, and the six to eight years it takes for the root to reach the size desired by Asian markets. He gets irked now when he finds sections of his thesis lifted in articles, and is proud that copies keep getting stolen from the Cornell library's shelves. His thesis also routinely disappears from the stacks of Greene County's public library. He likes to say it's poached.

BEFORE WE LEFT HIS office to go to the woods, a woman entered carrying a glass jar. She was a client—that's extension-speak for *county resident with a problem.* The jar in her hands contained a bug, and she wanted to know what it was. She complained that they had gotten inside her house and become a nuisance. Beyfuss told her it was a black vine beetle, usually found on rhododendrons. He nosed around the piles of papers for a book with a passage about the black vine beetle, pulled on cerulean-blue-framed reading glasses, and read it aloud. Then he photocopied the page for her. His professional recommendation: Squish the bugs.

Few of the county's residents these days rely on farming, or need advice from farm agents like Beyfuss. Since the turn of the twentieth century, he explained as we drove out along the ridges west of Cairo, Greene County's population has shrunk by half. Most of the farms are now owned by people who don't live there. Forests have recovered from near-leveling early in the 1900s; now they cover almost 90 percent of the county. Nature has made this stretch of the Catskills very desirable to millionaires, and magazines have dubbed the area "the new Hamptons."

Speculative buying by the wealthy has sent property taxes through the roof. Every week, Beyfuss would get another call from a farmer desperate to make his or her land (mostly old dairy pastures and wood lots) productive enough to cover the taxes. That's why Beyfuss became an advocate of growing "simulated-wild" ginseng, the awkward term for a practice that mainly consists of laying down seeds lightly in a forest, covering them and leaving them alone. Beyfuss figured that the high value of this nearly-wild ginseng (not truly wild, because someone put the seeds there) could help farmers make enough money after eight years to keep their land under forest cover. But the residents who came to Beyfuss in desperation could rarely wait eight years to turn a profit. He had to reach them earlier. He had tried different ways, including a column in local papers and a weekly TV show on Sunday mornings. "Kids across the county hated me," he said, "because their cartoons didn't start until I was off." He tried getting the word out in compendiums, too; for the *Encyclopedia of New York State,* he boiled down his years of accumulated wisdom on ginseng into a haikulike compression of one page. He struggled with that distillation for months.

Beyfuss was not introducing a radical idea. Ginseng has haunted the Catskills for centuries. He pointed, through his windshield, to a green knob in the distance, known as Ginseng Mountain. That was how it was designated when these hills were given names on maps in the early 1800s. The name recalls a time when ginsenging expeditions went into the woods for days at a time and returned with many sacks full of root to sell.

Back then, you could almost make a career digging ginseng. In 1837, residents of one remote valley in western North Carolina pulled 86,000 pounds of ginseng root out of the ground. That's roughly twenty large wagonloads, or a small house filled up to eye-level with roots, estimates Gary Kauffman, a botanist with the Forest Service. Go back to 1800 and you find that ginseng was established as the United States' first major export to the Far East. Rewind further back into the empires of France and England, and you find the two superpowers in the 1700s battling over ginseng and furs in North American forests.

There's not much ginseng on Ginseng Mountain anymore. The name drew generations of diggers and they mined it out. (In 1889 *The New York Times* reported that large quantities of big roots were still being dug in the Catskills and sold for what, in 2004, would be over sixty-two dollars a pound.) There are still a few old-timers in Greene County who know how to collect the root and sell it, but they are increasingly rare.

Women diggers have always been rare, Beyfuss said, even though women make better diggers. "Girls are better at finding ginseng than guys," he said. He speculated that women may be more observant.

Ginsenging traditions remain stronger further south, in Appalachia. For one thing, Beyfuss said, digging wild ginseng doesn't pay people in this area a wage comparable to what they could find in the city not so far away. Then there's the climate. "Our winters are ferocious. People get the hell out of here." Maybe you could survive winter in a tar-sided shack in the West Virginia woods, but here—due east of Buffalo—that's just not possible. Yet Beyfuss hoped that with simulated-wild ginseng, he could help revive a New York tradition in which families supplemented their income with native species from local forests, in ways more ecologically sound than conventional dairy farms, which invest a great deal of energy, resources, and antibiotics to grow animals that are not well suited to these hill slopes.

The ginseng festival, he believed, might rekindle interest among old-timers and spark curiosity among a group that he called "new down-homers": people who grew up nearby, moved to the city for work, and later returned to the countryside. Beyfuss knew the obstacles to making ginseng more profitable, which include layers of middlemen and the fact that consumers lack good information about the value of locally grown ginseng. But he also saw possibilities: a huge market familiar with ginseng's use as a tonic lay in the city just a few hours down the Hudson, but many of those people didn't know that ginseng grew in forests so close to them. So he printed his festival handbills, posted them all through the city's Chinese and Korean neighborhoods, and waited.

BY THE TIME WE left the car at the roadside and hiked into the woods for the first ginseng foray of the season, it was a warm late morning on the way to hot. *Hunt* struck me as a strange term to apply to a plant, but ginseng doesn't just sit there like other plants. According to legends on both sides of the Pacific, ginseng retreats from view. It camouflages itself, or stays underground, dormant, still as a stone, for several years in a row before sending up a stalk. "Ginseng is the tiger of the plant world," begins a report by TRAFFIC International, a watchdog organization that monitors endangered species. One grower, a former accountant with decades of hard-nosed farming experience, would talk about ginseng as if it had human qualities. "In the spring," he said, "if they think the year's going to be crummy, they won't grow. They'll just lie dormant." He caught himself and said of course plants don't think, *people* think. All the same, he insisted that ginseng could sense weather months in advance and respond to it.

Beyfuss, too, was intrigued by the way that ginseng plants go dormant, apparently for years at a time. The root doesn't die, but stays in a kind of suspended animation. Then another year it will send up a shoot. This unpredictability has caused people to watch ginseng very closely.

As we ducked under a barbed-wire fence, Beyfuss explained that in New York ginseng season starts September 1, but often harvesters will go a few weeks early to scout out patches. For confusing historical reasons, the government lumps ginseng with fish and wildlife, not plants. Every year, the Office of Scientific Authority in the U.S. Fish and Wildlife Service assesses the demographics of wild American ginseng in the eastern states and decides what controls to put on its export. Each of the nineteen states that exports ginseng runs its own program of registering buyers and recording how much ginseng they purchase from diggers. States have imposed a hunting season on ginseng collection. That season varies from state to state, and not with great consistency. You might expect the season to start earlier in the north, where the fall comes first, and later in the south. Nope. Tennessee's season starts two weeks before New York's.

Beyfuss was a friend of the man in whose woods we were foraging. The land was relatively low-lying, almost too damp to support ginseng. We continued downhill through maples and clusters of hemlock. The underbrush was sparse where the shade was heaviest. Ginseng likes shade. A dry stream bed angled along at our left. Beyfuss crossed over.

Standing on top of a berm on the far side, he inhaled.

"Smells like ginseng habitat," he said. "I don't know what it is, but I know that smell." I couldn't tell if he was hamming or sincere—all I smelled was the warm scent of decomposing wood and leaves—but there was no denying that Beyfuss knew this terrain like an old lover. And his claim on the place felt more intimate than science. In fact, he denied any scientific authority. "I'm just walking around the woods," he said, referring all questions about science to the Forest Service botanists. No, Beyfuss prowled the woods more like an old ginseng hunter.

Poaching is a common problem among ginsengers, but Beyfuss drew a line between poaching and theft. Theft, of course, was wrong. Theft involved taking something from someone who was obviously planning to use it. By contrast, poaching meant illegally using a natural resource that nobody else was planning to use. Intent plays a major role in this distinction. If you posted signs declaring GINSENG: KEEP OUT!, Beyfuss insisted that would help you make a legal case for treating any trespasser as a felon, because the signs show you know the value of what you have. His distinction between theft and poaching dovetailed nicely with his own past, which included digging ginseng on land whose owner didn't know the plant was there.

We had the woods to ourselves. He pointed out plants that signal ginseng territory: baneberry, another light shrubby plant called black cohosh, and jack-in-the-pulpit, a low-lying flower with red berries like ginseng's. "Fool's ginseng" is a good impostor, except that the leaflets don't all start from the same point on the stem; it's sarsaparilla. Other plants look like ginseng, too: Virginia creeper, hickory seedlings, and occasionally poison ivy. (Poison-ivy hives are a ginsenger's occupational hazard.) We passed hemlock and pines, partridgeberry, herb Robert, doll's eye, maidenhair fern, false Solomon seal, yellow-topped boletus mushrooms. Beyfuss picked a handful of mushrooms to use at home for seasoning meals.

This landscape had attracted him ever since he was a kid in Jersey City. In visits to his uncle's dairy farm, Beyfuss decided early on (at the age of four, he claims) that one day he would live here. Soon he was working summers on the farm.

"By the time I was sixteen I'd grown to hate cows," he told me, a furtive confession for an agriculture agent. From the dairy farm he switched to a horse farm. After graduating from Rutgers, he got jobs shoeing horses, working at gas stations, cleaning toilets at a factory in Schenectady. In 1976, when he got married and needed a steady job, the county posted an announcement for an assistant extension agent. He took that job and has been there through two marriages, two kids, and twenty-five 'sang seasons.

Suddenly, standing amid stinging nettle and blackberry prickers, he knelt down. There it was. "Four prong," he said.

This ginseng plant, he estimated, was fifteen to twenty years old. We studied it without a word. This was the first ginseng of the season, and its ordinary appearance made me pause. It was indeed a four-prong, with several clusters of leaves off the central stem—a good-size buck in ginseng terms—but it did not stand out markedly from the shrubs and the jack-in-the-pulpits nearby. Yet we were in a ginseng patch.

"The more you look, the more you see," Beyfuss said. Almost immediately, he pointed out another, just a bare stem. Although deer had nibbled off the leaves (deer and wild turkey love ginseng), Beyfuss could identify the plant by its central stem and the remaining bracts.

I had been thinking that by the end of that fall, I would be able to find the plant in the wild by myself. A century ago that would have been easy: ginseng patches grew thick with sprouts that multiplied from a granddaddy, enough so that one patch could yield a hundred pounds of root. But those days were gone. Now I wondered if my goal was reasonable. I have loved wandering in the woods since I was a kid, but I'm not patient enough to find a needle in a haystack.

Beyfuss had hunted ginseng throughout its range, which at one point stretched to the eastern edge of Nebraska and down into Florida, although reports of it in the Sunshine State have been disputed. He could reel off the regional names it had sprouted: "We call it ginseng or jin shang or 'sang. Down South, they call it 'sang or 'seng. In the Midwest, they call it shang." As you go south through the plant's native range, down the Alleghenies through the Appalachians to Georgia, the indicator plants change, too. Blue cohosh gives way to black cohosh. But core terms like *prong* remain the same.

Despite his obvious passion for the plant, Beyfuss showed restraint as a digger. Even though it was in season now, he merely pointed out the ginseng to me and moved on. He wanted to keep these patches intact. "It makes me nervous that I'm not seeing any babies here," he said, scanning one patch where the demographics weren't right. "This is the third year in a row that I haven't seen them." A responsible digger, he will spread ginseng berries around to germinate and assure another generation. He didn't harvest much wild root anymore. After all, he had a lot of simulated-wild ginseng on his own land. And although he had a dealer's license, he didn't sell much. At this point in his career, Beyfuss' main quarry was the plant's odd habits, like the dormancy phenomenon.

Beyfuss knew a digger who was walking across a pasture one day and, right in the middle of the field, found a ginseng patch. Given the plant's habitat, this is like finding a skateboarder on the eighth green of an exclusive private golf course. Its appearance in that open field made the digger question the pasture's history, so he did some research. Ten years before becoming a pasture, it was a meadow; ten years before it became a meadow, it was underwater in a pool dammed by beavers. The digger decided that the ginseng plants must have been submerged by the dam with a suddenness that virtually pickled them. When the dam broke, the soil resurfaced just as suddenly, leaving ginseng *en pleine air.*

SEVERAL YEARS AGO BEYFUSS launched an effort to collect American ginseng seeds everywhere the plant is native. That requires tromping the woods in almost every state east of the Mississippi and a few to the west as well, although in many of those states it's exceedingly rare. So far he has taken samples from New York, Pennsylvania, Ohio (where he'd gathered seeds just a few weeks earlier), Kentucky, Tennessee, West Virginia, and North Carolina. He was planning trips to Illinois, Indiana, Wisconsin, and Michigan. Soon he would be rummaging around Maine, New Jersey, Massachusetts, Vermont, Minnesota, and South Carolina. He paused at New Hampshire: "I could probably find it there but it's going to be work." (There's also a state law there against collecting wild ginseng.) And he was sure that ginseng grows wild somewhere in Connecticut, probably behind a big suburban estate. He also located a source on the outskirts of Washington, D.C. "I've got to see if she can find some ginseng in Maryland," he mused. "That will be a trick."

His original plan was to collect all the native varieties so that he could cross-breed a "truly American ginseng," but that changed. He didn't see noticeable differences among plants from the various regions. Plants from Ohio seeds looked a lot like plants grown from New York stock. A Cornell colleague conducted

DNA analyses that showed that genotypically, too, Beyfuss's seeds from various provenances were as varied—and as alike—as any two plants within the same population. (Beyfuss tells people that he scrapes together a thousand dollars a year to collect the seed, while his coworker in the Cornell lab gets fourteen times that amount to run the DNA analyses.) It seemed to him that ginseng expresses genetic traits as randomly as apples, which are notoriously unstable. Others disputed this, but Beyfuss was convinced that there is no truly wild American ginseng anywhere, that all the ginseng in forests across North America was fostered by centuries of people putting seed back in the soil; that even the most remote ginseng patch has had some human contact, however deep in the distant past.

Then what's the point of collecting all that seed? If there are no longer any native populations, why bother foraging for seed in forests everywhere as if there were? He gave two reasons: first, to prove himself wrong (a.k.a. the null hypothesis). If populations across the native range really do vary, he wants to know. Second, he wanted to have representatives of the full range available for further genetic studies. He has planted his stash of all his selections at two discrete locations several hours' drive apart.

Beyfuss still found it hard to describe why, exactly, ginseng merits all this treatment. "What is ginseng good for?" he asked, and then answered himself: "Everything, and not really anything." In Chinese medicine it's an all-purpose tonic, often blended with more toxic herbs to mellow their effect. In Western medicine it's gaining converts for relieving severe fatigue. Doctors at New York City's prestigious Sloane-Kettering hospital have prescribed American ginseng to help cancer patients cope with the stresses of chemotherapy and radiation treatment. It's a medically respected herb, he said, and there's a great demand for it.

With the few wild ginseng roots that he does collect, and several other herbs, Beyfuss makes a small private line of Doctor Bob's medicinals. The Doctor Bob line includes a cough medicine made from colt's foot, *Tussilago farfara*. There's also Doctor Bob's Mullein, a tobacco made from the leaves of *Verbascum*, a tall, spiky plant that grows in the stream bed we passed. Then there's Doctor Bob's Ginseng Elixir, which he makes by taking old roots, at least fifty years old, and extracting them in Everclear. "You know Everclear?" he said with a bad-boy grin. He immerses the root in the pure grain alcohol, waits until the liquid turns golden, and decants it. Then he mixes it with grape juice, apple juice, and maple syrup. (It actually doesn't taste that bad.) Then there's Doctor Bob's ginseng berry wine.

At that point, imagining the combination of ginseng bitterness with the sourness of homemade wine, I nearly gagged.

Beyfuss admitted that it tasted terrible. The year before he took thirteen pounds of ginseng berries and fermented them "the way you make any fruit wine." It had quite a kick. As he started talking about how you can smoke Verbascum, I remembered my mother asking me hesitantly, "Can you get high from ginseng?" People have tried. My wife tried to smoke ginseng back in high school. Talking with Beyfuss, that question hovered in the air. He started describing Doctor Bob's ginseng berry wine, and I realized the man lives for the adrenaline rush of his interest in the plant more than the plant itself. Unlike most ginseng manufacturers, Doctor Bob makes only modest claims for his products.

We crawled under the rusty barbed wire and walked back to the road nearly empty-handed, except for the boletus mushrooms that Beyfuss held between splayed fingers. We passed back into grassland along a pond's edge. Closing his friend's outer gate behind us, he explained why he's not interested in testing cropping combinations or companion plants that could possibly make simulated-wild ginseng more profitable. "Ginseng's the only one I care about," he said frankly. "The others are just plants. Ginseng's special."

Pressed to explain why, words failed him. He can't articulate the feeling he gets from hunting shang, he said, except to say that it "reinforces the primeval connection between humans and plants." For Beyfuss, ginseng's mystery defies rational thought.

We crossed the road and re-entered the everyday world, stopping in a driveway to retrieve a fertilizer spreader for his friend. The magic was already fading. You could tell, as Beyfuss settled into the car, that the rest of the day would be routine. The first hunt of the season was done.

TWO

The Doctors Debate

Of all the panaceas, adaptogens, and tonics,
the "gold standard" is ginseng.

—Walter H. Lewis and Memory P. Elvin-Lewis,
Medical Botany, 2003

Americans now spend well over $100 million a year on items that list ginseng as an ingredient, ranging from dietary supplements, teas, and lozenges to facial scrubs and ointments. The brands on supermarket shelves have, in a few years, grown as varied as genres in a music store: there's New Age (Gaia Herb, Garden of Life brands), folk (Traditional Medicinals), country (Country Life), and heavy-metal counterparts (Ginseng Powermax 4x and Siberian Sport 5000). Even venerable One-a-Day has adapted, with its Energy Formula that combines American ginseng with B-vitamins.

Ginseng's popularity is part of a larger surge in Americans' consumption of herbal foods and beverages: from $20 million in 1997 to over a billion dollars a year now. This trend caused concern at the U.S. Food and Drug Administration, and in 2001 it warned companies that some products with "novel ingredients" like ginseng could be illegal.

In the face of this seismic change, it's understandable why consumer advocates and medical skeptics are leery of ginseng root and the claims made for it. An assessment by Nutrition Action Newsletter in 1999 said that ginseng products had the worst track record of mislabeling of any popular supplement; 15 percent of the purported ginseng products they tested contained no ginseng at all. Soon after that, a report by Consumer Lab found that less than half of the ginseng products tested contained even a threshold level of 2 percent ginsenosides, the active chemical compounds in ginseng. Worse, many of the products in their test were contaminated by pesticides or heavy metals (elements such as mercury, arsenic, and lead that can cause damage at low concentrations); eight had high levels of the pesticides quintozene and hexachlorobenzene, which are potential carcinogens, and two contained high concentrations of lead—over three micrograms per daily serving. Finding a true health supplement on retail shelves was no easy task. Manufacturers have since begun to improve their reliability in response to wary consumers.

Besides false labeling, skeptics hold a second, deeper layer of distrust of the root itself. Stacks of clinical trial results have so far failed to clarify the exact action of ginseng in the body. Some nutritionists state flatly that ginseng doesn't work, and that Asian ginseng, the more studied of the two, doesn't boost energy levels or memory and doesn't reduce stress. A visit to www.quackwatch.org, a website dedicated to exposing medical fraud and bad advice, reveals an equally adamant stance. Dr. Stephen Barrett, the website's editor and vice president of the National Council Against Health Fraud, is a retired psychiatrist and an aggressive watchdog who has tracked the literature for over a quarter century. He has said he has yet to find a mail-order health product that lives up to its claims, and remains skeptical about ginseng's benefits. In his article "Why Quackery Sells," ginseng appears alongside such suspects as aromatherapy, bee pollen, and pyramids as products hawked with a series of quack arguments. One example is the idea that everyone's body chemistry is slightly different, and therefore the FDA's Recommended Dietary Allowances don't apply. Barrett also becomes suspicious when people say a product is part of a philosophical conflict or paradigm shift. These arguments have indeed been used to explain why ginseng's value in Asian medicine has not been clearly validated by Western clinical research.

Yet interest in ginseng and other natural products continues to grow among Western physicians as well, many of whom have grown frustrated with the limitations of conventional allopathic medicine and concerned by the mounting costs of its treatments. Their interest shows the lines are not as clear-cut as quack versus physician, or science versus superstition, or even East versus West. What explains this ongoing ferment?

Some experts say it all goes back to Nixon—the misinformation, the distrust. Skeptics and proponents both point to the moment when Richard Nixon opened the door for U.S. relations with China in the early 1970s as a landmark event. The skeptics say that started a fractured relationship with the truth; the advocates say it opened Western awareness to alternative ways of healing. Three decades later, American medical opinion on ginseng's healing properties remains divided.

• • •

PROBABLY THE MOST IN-DEPTH comparison of Western medicine and Chinese medicine came near the end of the twentieth century in a posthumous publication by Joseph Needham, a distinguished biochemistry researcher in England. Needham is recognized as the first director of the natural sciences department in the United Nations Educational, Scientific and Cultural Organization. (Biographers say that he put the *S* in UNESCO.) At the age of forty, Needham gave up biochemistry research, in which he was moving toward a chemical explanation for embryonic development. Instead, he embarked on a second career studying Chinese science and medicine. This change was triggered by meeting three young Chinese students at Cambridge, one of whom would eventually become his wife. Needham spent the next forty years of his life compiling a seventeen-volume opus, *Science and Civilisation in China.* At one point in that exhaustive assessment, he drew up a balance sheet tallying the merits and weaknesses of both medical systems.

Particularly since the discovery of penicillin and other antibiotics, Western medicine's great strength has been in the treatment of acute diseases, Needham concluded. Chinese medicine, on the other hand, has a long history of clinical experience in relieving painful but less-acute conditions, like arthritis, that have resisted successful treatment in Western medicine. Another strength of Chinese medicine, Needham wrote, lay in two core concepts: the view of the healthy body as a balanced system, and the idea that disease is a process with different stages. Both Eastern and Western systems had weaknesses. Western medicine's focus on single-chemical medications could involve serious side effects, and too often failed to consider the body as a whole. The main weakness of Chinese medicine was that its theories had adapted little to our improved understanding of the body's chemistry and physiology. Needham viewed the two systems as complementary parts of a puzzle, and saw that this posed an opportunity to create a powerful new medical approach that would draw on the best of both traditions. The question was how and when this fusion would happen.

THE BOTTLES OF CAPSULES ON supermarket shelves don't look like promising forerunners of the synthesis that Needham envisioned, but health innovations have grown from lowly beginnings. Experimenting with plants has traditionally been an inelegant science. The father of herbal medicine in China, Shen Nong, would ingest leaves and roots as part of his testing method. A legendary emperor also known as the "Divine Farmer," Shen Nong reportedly lived around 2000 BC and compiled the first compendium of herbal medicines and their uses. He is said to have discovered and personally tested Asian ginseng, as well as rhubarb (*Rheum* species) and cinnamon *(Cinnamomum aromaticum)*. By 225 BC, his compendium, known as *The Divine Farmer's Classic of Materia Medica,* was famous. From that earliest written record, ginseng was important for maintaining a person's *qi* (pronounced "chi"), the vital energy at the heart of Taoist medicine.

The *Materia Medica* fused empirical experience with herbs and the emerging philosophy of Taoism, which looked to nature for clues on how to live. The Taoists realized that nature contained all kinds of contradictions, so their system of mysticism included life's many contradictions as well. As one scholar wrote, "nothing, however strange it may be, is outside Nature."

The Taoists believed that by harmonizing the body's basic elements of male *(yang)* and female *(yin),* a person could maintain balance and prevent illness. "The best physicians always treat disease when it is not [yet] a disease," says the *Tao Te Ching,* or *Book of the Way.* "And so [their patients] are not ill." For Taoists, the idea of giving drugs to a sick person was like waiting until you're thirsty to dig a well. Wasn't that too late?

Asian ginseng's reputation as a mild stimulant fit well with the Taoist idea of maintaining the body's qi: when people nibbled at ginseng, they seemed to feel more energy. Described as sweet and cool—not too potent or toxic—it was mild enough to combine well with other herbs. Plus, its shape corresponded with another Taoist idea, that humans mirror the universe around them. (Early medical encyclopedias made this literal, saying that objects in nature could help cure their counterpart in the human body. That's why walnuts were good for the brain.) The resemblance between an odd, branchy ginseng root and the human form made ginseng promising for many human ills. The name *ginseng* stems from the Cantonese term for "image of man."

The Taoist view of balance spans medicine and philosophy, with qi at its core. Chinese philosophy, like the Bible, holds that the world started from a "block of chaos," in the words of Paul Hsu, one of the largest dealers in American ginseng. "Qi made that move into yin and yang. Qi means what? Power. Movement." The big bang of qi.

• • •

THESE CONCEPTS RESOUND MORE clearly against a forest backdrop than they do in a laboratory. In fact, a temple forest grove in Thailand introduced me to Taoism. There a tree with a handwritten placard nailed to its trunk offered a passage from Chuang Tzu and its final, startling contradiction:

> The man in whom Tao acts without impediment does not struggle to make money and does not make a virtue of poverty. He goes his way without relying on others and does not pride himself on walking alone. . . . He is not always looking for right and wrong, always deciding "Yes" or "No." The ancients said: The man of Tao remains unknown. Perfect virtue produces nothing. No-self is trueself. And the greatest man is "Nobody."

These ideals of independent thought, nonjudgmental observation, and humility come naturally when surrounded by soaring teak trees or ancient, gnarled oaks.

In another forest, a different interpreter of the Tao appeared in Syl Yunker, a ginseng grower from Kentucky. Yunker, aged seventy-three, was leading a group on a brisk walk in Virginia's Blue Ridge mountains. Yunker had absorbed Taoist teachings while living in Asia, and spoke of ginseng in terms of balance and energy, but made no claim to medical authority. He was more down-to-earth. He took a bit of ginseng root between his gum every day, and when he went hunting 'sang he carried a crossbow to scare off poachers. As we walked in the woods, he explained his view of the relationship between American ginseng and Asian ginseng.

By reputation, Asian ginseng is "hot" and a greater stimulant than American ginseng, which many regard as "cool." This polarity became exaggerated in the 1800s, possibly due to geography. Asian ginseng came from the cold climes of northeastern China, Korea, and Siberia and seemed to be in contrast with those wintry origins. American ginseng came into China from the subtropical port of Canton, where people wanted it to cool them off. So American roots were yin, and Asian roots were yang.

Yunker said these distinctions might also indicate the different character of the two cultures. He calls ginseng an *adaptogen* (a word from Chinese medicine that refers to plants that help the body with everyday adjustments) and uses the term broadly. "Look at the cultures," he said. "Americans are all stressed out. They need to slow down." American ginseng, which contains more calmative ginsenosides, is suited for that. "In China, under the bureaucracy of fifty years of communism, everybody's bored. They're looking for excitement." So they turn to Asian ginseng as a stimulant.

THE DIFFERENCES BETWEEN THE two types of ginseng are less important than similarities in how they react with qi, and their shared classification as adaptogens. Chinese medicine categorizes herbs by their nature, taste, configuration, color, and physical properties. An herbalist combines herbs into a formula for a particular mix of properties that suit the diagnosis and understanding of the body's systems. Like the Divine Farmer's *Materia Medica,* later Chinese medical texts described ginseng as a plant that nourishes or tonifies qi, particularly for the heart organs. Deficiency of qi, for example, is common among elderly people with chronic heart disease who suffer from cold arms and legs, and shortness of breath. (It can correspond to a form of angina in Western medical diagnostics.) For qi deficiency, ginseng might be prescribed together with herbs that warm the body and eliminate dampness. Different herbs are used when the need is to expel excess qi, tonify moisture, or build blood.

Alongside the classical texts of the pharmacopoeia, Chinese medicine progressed through "lineages" of clinical practice. The clinical experience continued to grow through these lines of training, apprenticeship, and physicians' case studies, long after the conceptual framework behind Chinese medicine stopped evolving. The case studies were often extremely detailed about symptoms and procedures used with each patient, and as subtle in their arguments about diagnoses and treatments as Western research articles. They described formulas as combinations of leading and supporting ingredients, a hierarchy that designated each herb in the formula as a ruler, minister, assistant, or envoy. One formula that combined mild herbs for tonifying qi was known as the Four Gentlemen (the name comes from a Confucian term for an exemplar of ideal behavior). Besides Asian ginseng *(ren shen),* the other three gentlemen were *bai zhu* *(Atractylodis macrocephalae,* or Largehead Atractylodes), *fu ling* *(Sclerotium poriae cocos),* and *zhi gan cao* (honey-fried root of *Glycyrrhizae uralensis,* also called Chinese licorice).

In the late Song dynasty (AD 960–1279), Chen Ziming, a medical professor at an academy in Nanjing, criticized the misinformation that had grown up in earlier teachings and urged physicians to "search deeply for an all-round view." He re-evaluated ginseng and used it in his "Pills Better than Gold," which he prescribed for women recovering from childbirth. In that formula Chen used ginseng to stimulate qi and support white peony root, angelica and lovage rhizome, tree peony bark, and corydalis tuber, which all helped build blood.

Later in the Ming era (AD 1368–1644), Li Shizhen took up Chen's challenge and tackled the herculean task of distilling and organizing the accumulated knowledge of herbs, weeding out misinformation that had gathered over the centuries. Li devoted twenty-seven years to compiling his *Great Compendium of Herbs*. Published in 1596, after his death, it described ginseng as a mild, cool-natured tonic that "expresses the yang influence of spring" and that can be used to treat illnesses that affect both the upper and lower body. Li's work remains one of the definitive classical texts of herbal medicine. Experience with ginseng was growing more sophisticated, although the experts couldn't explain exactly how it worked.

As GINSENG'S USE BECAME increasingly canonized, its stock rose. Even beyond its health value, it gained a prestige worthy of the highest nobility. As early as 1274, Marco Polo had recounted for Europeans that ginseng was made into powders, teas, syrups, and a condiment for Asian dignitaries he visited in his travels. Then in the 1680s, a delegate of Louis XIV's ambassadorial mission to Siam (present-day Thailand), after conversations with other diplomats, became intrigued by this "treasure" and wrote back to Paris, "I have just learned . . . the method of using ginseng." He went on:

Its principal effect is to rectify blood and to return
strength to those who have lost it. One puts water in a
cup, makes it boil vigorously, throws in the roots of ginseng cut into small pieces, covers the cup well in order to
infuse the ginseng, and when the water cools, one takes
it in the morning before eating.

At the time, an epicurean sophistication was sweeping through
Europe, and Europeans were mad for new spices and flavors.
France was importing Asian herbs and foods and introducing
them to the rest of Europe with the urgency of a fashion craze,
so the envoy's message resonated in Paris. An exotic herb that also
offered health effects? That would be a double bonus. Soon Ital-
ian naturalist and physician Francesco Redi was gushing over
ginseng's benefits, saying that the tonic must be an ingredient in
any stew that repeals old age. (The word *tonic* itself gained currency around that time. The dictionary defines it as "something
that invigorates, restores, or refreshes," but a more specific usage,
going back to 1649, referred to anything that restores organs or
muscles to their normal, healthy condition.)

The French envoy, Abbé François-Timoléon de Choisy, a
playboy known for extravagant gambling and flamboyant trans-
vestite adventures, wrote a compelling account of Siamese life
and culture that became a bestseller back home. So when Siam
sent an ambassadorial mission to France in 1687, it stirred great
excitement.

The entourage docked in the harbor at Brest with a caravan
of gifts from the Siamese capital and an elaborate letter from the
Siamese king to Louis. The letter rested in a lavish gilt pyramid

that required eight guards to carry. The royal gifts included an array of lacquered tables, porcelains, silver sets, dishes for chocolates, and "a measure of eight taels of ginseng, placed in the hands of the ambassador himself," as well as a silver teapot for preparing the roots. (*Tael* is a traditional Chinese measure still used for weighing herbs and gold, one tael equaling three quarters of an ounce.) Ginseng, now an international symbol of good health and sophistication, had arrived on the global stage as the perfect thing for one cosmopolitan monarch to give another.

As the Siamese envoys took their procession from the coast to Paris, they were saluted at each village they passed with a royal fusillade. In Nantes, the local nobility lined up on horseback while the cannons boomed out the welcome. The whole country was abuzz over the exotic visitors. When they finally reached Paris, the exhausted diplomats were ushered to the grand palace at Versailles. Louis received them with great pomp in a state room, seated on his silver throne. In the formal ceremony, the Sun King expressed his deep appreciation for all their gifts, including the ginseng. Afterward he invited them to share in the kind of feast for which Versailles was famous, a "magnificent collation" of ragouts and other dishes. For years after that visit, French nobles sampled ginseng to revive flagging energy.

In America, interest in medicinal herbs often reflected trends from Europe, with cycles of high regard and acceptance followed by skepticism. In the late 1700s, China was recognized as a powerful and ancient empire, and its influence on Europeans' use of herbal remedies was at a peak. As a man of science, Benjamin Franklin followed these developments, and brought the first true Chinese rhubarb (used as a purgative) from London to Philadelphia for his friend, the naturalist John Bartram. A medical text of 1818 featured a drawing of American ginseng and described its use in China and Japan. The treatment was respectful if not embracing: ginseng's use in America was simply "as a demulcent in a few skin ointments," but the text noted that ginseng "has been one of the most important exports to China and other countries of the Far East." An 1836 encyclopedia of botanical medicines was more enthusiastic, saying there is "no reasonable doubt that the ginseng has really an invigorating and stimulant power when fresh." The *U.S. Pharmacopoeia* included ginseng in its list of herbs with therapeutic value for much of the nineteenth century, for use as a stimulant and a stomach medicine.

Early in the twentieth century, American use of medicinal herbs declined following the 1910 Flexner Report, a searing critique of medical education in the United States that influenced medical schools profoundly. The report urged that American medical schools focus on allopathic medicine, to the exclusion of many approaches that had once been popular, including herbalism.

As a result, most Americans didn't hear about Chinese herbal medicine again until the early 1970s, when growing popular interest in alternative lifestyles and traditions led to an exploration of other cultures and health systems. Chris Wanjek, who writes about health and medical misconceptions for *The Washington Post*, conducted an informal survey of health fads since that time and traced the rising interest in Chinese medicine back to Richard Nixon's trips to China. During an early diplomatic visit there, journalist James Reston was stricken with acute appendicitis and needed emergency surgery. With no time to consult Western doctors, Chinese physicians performed surgery, using acupuncture in lieu of anesthesia. Afterward Reston wrote accounts of his experiences with Chinese medicine for *The New York Times* and observed several more operations. Reston reported that even the surgeons "cannot agree on the theory of how the needle anesthesia works," and yet "they are operating on the pragmatic evidence and not waiting for theoretical justifications." The time was right for "serious medical exchange" between the two countries, he said.

Soon after that, Dr. Samuel Rosen, a physician with the Mount Sinai School of Medicine in New York, visited clinics in China and penned his own eyewitness account of acupuncture's benefits under the headline, "I Have Seen the Past and It Works." He wrote, "I have seen one of the most venerable arts in Chinese traditional medicine applied in the most modern of contexts in today's China." He described seeing an acupuncturist carefully locate target points on a patient's arm and insert needles that allowed the man to remain conscious and calm even as his chest was cut open for heart surgery. "I have no explanation for this phenomenon," Dr. Rosen conceded, "but science has no explanation for many observations that still elude investigation."

"Suddenly Chinese medicine was in the public eye," Wanjek told me. "I think it was at this point, in the 1970s, that Western medicine began to clash with Chinese medicine." The

American public wanted to know more, but Chinese medicine isn't easily adapted to clinical trials. It proceeds empirically and prescriptions vary, based on a patient's balance of characteristics. There was no way to plug Chinese acupuncture or whole-herb formulas into the standardized Western approach to clinical trials. Curious Americans fell back on hearsay.

Amid growing interest in finding alternatives to conventional medicine, many were intrigued by China's long-isolated culture, but they had no foundation for understanding it. Health news coverage of herbs became more hopeful and less cautious. In his informal survey, Wanjek found that articles on Chinese medicine were often upbeat and rather uncritical. Not until much later, when a pitcher for the Baltimore Orioles died from the Chinese herb ephedra in early 2003, did Wanjek see more critical reports about herbs. (Ultimately that death led to a ban on ephedra sales.) "In the United States, we have a caveman approach to herbs," he wrote in an e-mail. "Ginseng good; me take more ginseng. We add it to candy bars and sugary drinks. That can't be healthy."

OVER THE YEARS, ONE expert that both ginseng advocates and skeptics came to respect was Dr. Varro Tyler, a professor of pharmacology at Purdue University and a leading expert in pharmacognosy, the study of drugs from natural sources—plants, animals, and microorganisms. (An avid stamp collector, he also wrote a series of books about philatelic forgeries.) Tyler grew up in Nebraska, studied pharmacology at Yale and the University of Connecticut, and began to research local folk remedies while teaching at Purdue. His aim was to sift through remedies with a critical, scientific eye. This led him to travel throughout the country and abroad. His book, *Tyler's Honest Herbal,* first published in the early 1980s, provided a level-headed guide to the use of herbs. He reiterated his approach in a revised edition:

> Herbs are actually nothing more than diluted drugs. . . .
> They do not possess any magical or mystical properties,
> and like other drugs, they must be administered in proper
> doses for appropriate periods of time to produce their
> benefits. . . . As is the case with other drugs, the adminis-
> tration of herbs may produce undesirable side effects.

Tyler regarded ginseng warily. Although its botany and chemistry were reasonably well known, scientists still lacked a clear understanding of how—and if—ginseng worked. After reviewing the clinical research on both Asian and American ginseng since 1968, he concluded that "whatever pharmacological activity ginseng may possess is probably due mainly to its many chemical compounds, which are triterpenoid saponins." Those chemical compounds became commonly known as ginseno-sides. When scientists placed thin slivers of Asian and American ginsengs under the microscope with a solvent, they found a baker's dozen of these ginsenosides, to which they gave imaginative monikers: Ra, Rb, Rb_1, R_1, Rf, Rh_1, F_1, F_2, etc. They discovered that while ginsenosides were in all parts of the ginseng plant (roots, rhizomes, leaves and stems, and flowers), they tended to be more concentrated in the roots. Saponins react with water to make foam or lather; a number are used in detergents and emulsifiers. Ginseng's concentration of these saponins appeared to increase slightly as the plants got older. In the root, total saponin levels stepped up from 1.6 percent in the first year to 1.9 percent in the second, gradually increasing to the sixth year. The main differences between Asian and American ginsengs, it seemed, resulted from their different proportions of these ginsenosides.

The building blocks of its chemical makeup were becoming known and their effects were being tested in small animals, but how ginseng worked in the human body was a very different matter. In a revised edition of his book, Tyler noted clinical studies that indicated standardized ginseng extract appeared to promote a slightly improved quality of life—that is, a feeling of well-being and less fatigue. The revised edition was less skeptical about ginseng, but Tyler still doubted that the plant's activity could be proven until clinical trials were designed better for testing herbs, which contain too many compounds for conventional clinical studies to analyze well. In the 1990s, more clinical trials suggested that older people might benefit in varying degrees from a regimen of ginseng. Then in 1999, a series of monographs on herbal medicines authored by a German panel of experts was translated into English. These books, known as the Commission E monographs, evaluated the research literature on ginseng (along with three hundred other herbs) and approved it as a tonic for relieving extreme physical and mental fatigue, and for use in convalescence. The World Health Organization gave its own seal of approval for ginseng in a report released that same year.

In the summer of 2001 I spoke with Dr. Tyler to ask if recent research had changed his estimation of ginseng. He had retired, but at seventy-four remained very active in his field. He cited findings on ginsenosides that suggested some were stimulants, while others had a calmative or depressive effect on the central nervous system. (Rg_1 appeared to be a main stimulant, and Rb_1 a main calmative component. Recent research at the Baylor College of Medicine has suggested that Rb_1 and Rb_3 can slow brain-cell deterioration.) He was glad that the National Institutes of Health had taken up research that private industry had been unwilling to fund, and had established in 1998 a National Center for Complementary and Alternative Medicine, which funded a series of innovative experiments on ginseng and other herbs. Tyler applauded that effort and had few kind words for drug companies that refused to invest in research on herbs. "Frankly," he said, "I think some of the industrial firms have made a lot of money out of these herbal products and probably should put some of it back into research."

The studies that he found most impressive were conducted in St. Michael's Hospital in Toronto, on American ginseng's effect on adult-onset diabetes, also called type 2 diabetes. The Toronto researchers, led by Vladimir Vuksan, had published several papers that suggested that American ginseng, administered to a person within two hours before a meal, could help prevent the surge in blood sugar typically triggered by food. While that finding required further study, it showed promise for controlling such surges in diabetics.

Dr. Tyler remained doubtful of the sweeping claims made in ginseng's name, and skeptical that there was much difference between young and old roots. He repeated the need for standardization of how herbal extracts are made. But the word *tonic* had entered his vocabulary. "I think ginseng does have a tonic effect," he said. "As we learn more about these things our perceptions change, and I'm much less skeptical about ginseng than I was when I wrote that chapter." In his summary of the differences between American and Asian ginseng, he echoed Chinese medicine, but with a basis in science. Overall, he said, American ginseng had more calmative ginsenosides than Asian ginseng.

"If you're overwrought and you want to take ginseng to calm down a little bit, American ginseng may be your herb of choice," he told me. "If you need energy to pep up, then the Asian ginseng would be the herb of choice."

VARRO TYLER WAS A mentor for Dr. Mary Hardy, the medical director of the Integrative Medicine Medical Group at the Cedars-Sinai Medical Center in Los Angeles. They traveled together to the Amazon to study how medicinal plants were used there, and he continued to share his experience through the years, answering her questions and pointing out new developments. Hardy also studied with traditional Eastern herbalists. Having grown up in New Orleans, a fifth-generation physician and the granddaughter of a Louisiana family doctor, she has always been an independent thinker, fascinated by a wide range of medical practice. Her thumbnail metaphor for the relationship between Western and Eastern approaches is that Western medicine acts as the head and Eastern medicine is the heart. Western medicine follows a linear, analytical approach to how medicine works; Eastern medicine focuses more on the relationships within the body's systems. Each tells you something useful.

"In Chinese medicine there's a functional approach," she told me. "So ginseng activity occurs in a formula; it occurs in a functional context."

Hardy, who talks faster than anyone I have ever met, came face-to-face with Chinese medicine during her residency at Tufts University's New England Medical Center, on the edge of Boston's Chinatown. There she was a primary-care provider for the community, and her patients were mainly unassimilated Chinese who had come to Boston from Hong Kong. Older patients would arrive at the clinic without an interpreter, and a routine examination would turn into a major challenge. Hardy made flashcards with various phrases ("Good morning." "Hello, I'm the doctor." "Point to where it hurts.") and asked a social worker to translate them into Chinese. Hardy would hold these up one at a time for her patients. Sometimes she would hold up a card that said, "May I examine you?" and wave her stethoscope around. The women's responses gave her an unexpected lesson in cultural exchange.

"They would roll back their cuffs, they'd unbutton two buttons around their navel, and they'd stick out their tongue," Hardy told me. "I was like, 'I think I'm missing something.'"

The need to understand her patients pushed Hardy out into the neighborhood. She talked with people and visited the local grocery and herb shops, where she encountered ginseng. She walked into Chinese pharmacies and asked about the products and what they cost. Older ginseng roots sold for two hundred dollars each. This raised other questions for her. Slowly she came to understand the context for how ginseng is used in Chinese medicine.

Hardy finds an analogy in the language. Chinese doesn't have a past tense in the way that English does; an event's location in time is understood by looking at the whole phrase. A modifier like *yesterday* or *tomorrow* places the event in its context. In the same way, she said, Chinese physicians use ginseng in the context of improving quality of life. That's an elusive concept for Western medicine, which prefers absolute quantitative measures. She found just a few Western studies that assessed improved quality of life from ginseng use. One paper in the *Annals of Pharmacotherapy* found that Asian ginseng enhanced aspects of mental health and social functioning after four weeks of use. (On the other hand, the incidence of adverse effects for ginseng users was higher than for the placebo group.) In another study, researchers at Connecticut's Hartford Hospital concluded that ginseng use may have improved "various facets of Quality of Life," although the overall improvements were slight.

Gradually Hardy moved toward a medical practice that combined Eastern and Western approaches. She traveled to China with a group of doctors in April 1982, when the country was still closed and it was very difficult for foreigners to get around. In hospital pharmacies she watched technicians prepare herbal medicines for prescriptions. Behind a bank of glass, they stood before cabinets of wooden drawers, measuring out combinations of roots and leaves, and scribbling instructions for the patients on how to cook the mixture at home. Hardy saw that a lot of those pharmacy cabinets contained ginseng.

During that trip Hardy fell ill with what a Western doctor would probably diagnose as a fungal lung infection, caused by the dust storms that blow through Beijing every spring. She was with a group of physicians, so all her tour mates had suggestions of what she should take. "I was like, 'Hell no! I'm going to go to the Chinese doctors.'" Hardy was diagnosed as having excess heat in the lung, and given an herbal solution.

"It was *hideous*," she said. "But I got much better. Then I left it on the plane. And I relapsed, and I was sick as a dog for a month."

Years later, Hardy returned to China. It was her turn to surprise her hosts. She gave a talk at Beijing's Guanamen Traditional Chinese Medicine Hospital on her use of Asian ginseng as a single herb to help relieve the extreme fatigue of cancer patients undergoing chemotherapy. She knew her audience of Chinese physicians might use ginseng as a cancer prophylactic, but never during treatment. Their response to her presentation was immediate and blistering. "You can't give this to patients with cancer! It's too hot! It will promote growth!' Blah, blah, blah. They just went nuts, totally nuts." Her audience reacted with as much outrage as American doctors might have registered at the idea of sticking needles into their patients. Working between two medical systems seemed to ensure attacks from both sides.

For Hardy and other physicians who would like to see Western medicine integrate ginseng into its practice, three main priorities are: better understanding of the herb's uses (both traditional and modern), good quality control for products, and better education of patients. She is leery of ginseng's commercial bandwagon and does not recommend products on health-store shelves. She prefers to work with experienced herbalists, but that, too, depends on the individual herbalist and their training. Since most people don't have ready access to well-trained herbalists, Hardy believes that what is needed is a combination of traditional and modern systems.

To GET A CLOSER PERSPECTIVE on Chinese medicine, I consulted a listing of licensed New York Chinese herbalists and made an appointment with Susan Eng in midtown Manhattan. For Eng, the tension between Eastern and Western medicine is a family affair. Her father was a Western-trained doctor who had little use for terms like "qi deficiency." He had studied in Hong Kong and received his medical license there before the family emigrated to the United States on New Year's Eve, 1972. He wanted one of his children to become a Western doctor, but Susan resisted. She loved medicine but not Western medicine.

"When I was born, I was very, very sick," she explained. "My godmother nursed me back to health with herbs. So in the back of my mind, I always wanted to study herbology."

Eng dutifully got an undergraduate degree from Yale, but then, as she describes it, found her way back. She completed the program in acupuncture and herbology at the Pacific College of Oriental Medicine, on Broadway, and apprenticed with a clinician before getting her certification.

A member of the American Association of Oriental Medicine, Eng's practice was located in an airy office building on Thirty-first Street. Her reception area resembled any doctor's office, but inside the door was pasted a cartoon. It showed a mastodon with spears sticking out of its butt, as caveman hunters closed in. A thought balloon from the mastodon said: "That's odd. My neck suddenly feels better." The caption read "Early acupuncture."

Eng met me in the reception area with the relaxed, confident voice of a therapist or a good deejay. Her office had the standard examining table covered in a white paper sheet. Her diagnostic procedure starts with questions, asking about all aspects of a patient's health to learn what that person's usual balance is, and any "pattern of imbalance or disharmony" that has concerned them. To treat a woman with unusually cold hands or feet, for example, Eng would ask about the patient's energy, her appetite, her stools. Loose stools might signal a deficiency of qi or yang. Americans are often embarrassed to discuss their bowel movements. "A lot of people are not so aware of their bodies," Eng said. "They'll say, 'I've never thought about this.'" After those questions Eng makes her own observations, checking the patient's tongue, stomach, and pulse.

Taking the pulse is more complex than merely counting off a minute's worth of arterial surges. Eng took both of my wrists in her hands and worked three fingers on each wrist. The effect was like having someone fret each wrist like the neck of a guitar. The pulse on the right wrist told her about my qi and yang, while the left side indicated more about yin and the blood system. There are nine different pulse positions on each side, at different pressure levels beneath the skin.

Finally, after these questions and observations, Eng makes a diagnosis based on her experience and the classical medical texts. She admires those texts for the elegance of their treatments. "There are a few really beautiful classical formulas that use ginseng," she said. She mentioned the Four Gentlemen, and another formula that she uses often, *gui pi tang*. She wrote it out on a sheet of stationery, explaining that it helps with insomnia related to qi deficiency, which can involve fatigue and a digestive problem, like poor appetite. When qi doesn't flow well, that causes imbalance, ill health, and disease. If Eng identifies qi deficiency, blood deficiency, yang deficiency, or a combination of those, she prescribes ginseng with other herbs.

The thick book of the classical materia medica on her desk was a 1986 volume edited by two practitioners, Dan Bensky and Andrew Gamble. She had marked her copy with color tabs in green, yellow, blue, and red, with handwritten headings that would baffle most American doctors: Regulate Blood, Regulate Qi, Tonify Qi, Drain Dampness, Clear Heat, Calm Spirit, and Nourish Yin. Under the heading Tonify Qi, the first herb listed was ginseng. Problems with qi are most commonly found in the spleen and lungs, the main yin organs that extract qi from food and air. The text goes on to say that Asian ginseng is used for "severe collapsed qi conditions," that it benefits yin and generates fluids, and that wild roots from Jilin Province are best but are so expensive that they're used only in the gravest situations. Cultivated ginseng works fine and is cheaper. In fact, ginseng has nearly been priced out of clinical practice. Eng admitted that, depending on a patient's insurance and ability to pay, she may substitute a cheaper plant, like codonopsis, for the king of herbs.

Eng also made very clear that ginseng and other tonics are not always good for you. If qi is trapped in the stomach, for example, tonifying that qi would only make matters worse. She cited a case from her clinical apprenticeship of a patient who had taken huge doses of ginseng for years and had contracted liver damage. Rather than self-medicating, people should consult a trained herbalist.

When I voiced amazement that almost no English translation of the classical Chinese medical texts existed before 1986, Nixon raised his head again. For centuries, Eng reminded me, Chinese medicine interested only Chinese physicians. It gained broader popularity in the West, she said, only after Nixon traveled to China.

Eng's use of ginseng rigorously followed those medical texts, but the pressures of consumerism were evident in the Chinatown pharmacy where some of her prescriptions get filled. There, according to Tom Leung, a fourth-generation Chinese pharmacist and the pharmacy's manager, many people come in and simply buy ginseng without a prescription. Sometimes a patient insists that the pharmacist add items such as deer antler velvet or seahorses to a prescription, even though these are rarely mentioned in the medical texts. Leung likened this to someone asking their doctor for Prozac after seeing ads on television.

So his pharmacy sold both Asian and American ginseng, even though the classical texts were codified before Chinese physicians knew about the American species. Leung's supply of Asian ginseng came from a buyer in Shanghai who would wait for the price to go down, and then head into Anhui Province to collect a containerful. For American ginseng, Leung flew to Wisconsin with his uncle to buy shang from growers there. He would marvel at their farms, their big rough hands, and occasionally their awkwardness with business. It was as if they lived in different worlds, he said.

AFTER DECADES OF LIVING between two worlds, studying science and medicine in both West and East, the biochemist

Joseph Needham concluded that every medical system was bound by the culture where it developed. The ways that our medical systems gather knowledge are subtly shaped even by the languages we use. Still, he envisioned "an ecumenical medicine of the future," which would combine the clinical insights and techniques of Eastern medicine with a foundation in modern biology and physiology. That synthesis required people willing to take a hard look at the knowledge frameworks they inherited and to look beyond.

As clinical trial methodology advances and adapts to the complex compounds of whole herbs, ginseng might help nudge physicians toward such a synthesis. Then again, maybe that idea places too much weight on a small, gnarled root.

It was becoming clear, though, that ginseng's story involved much more than medical practice or malpractice. Another entry point stood just a few minutes' walk from Tom Leung's pharmacy.

THREE

The Emperor's Favorite

*Ginseng and sable skins are what our people
rely on for a livelihood.*

—HUANG TAIJI, Emperor of China (1592–1643)

ABOUT THREE TIMES A year, Bob Beyfuss makes the trip from the Catskills to Manhattan's Chinatown.

"I love Chinatown," he says. "I love Manhattan. And I always like to bring a few ginseng roots down and eat really good." He uses his own roots to promote New York–grown ginseng in Chinatown herb shops like Tom Leung's.

The city has changed since Beyfuss was a teenager taking the subway from Jersey City: some neighborhoods have shrunk, others revived. "Little Italy is about a half a block now, to be honest," he says. "You've got Forlini's, Umberto's, two or three other restaurants, a bakery, a cheese store, which is now run by Chinese people, and that's it. The rest of Little Italy has been swallowed by Chinatown. Chinatown's still very cool."

Beyfuss relishes the energy of walking in the city and the thrill of a bargain. Not sidewalk-vendor haggling, but a more basic barter. He likes a deal that takes place more through gestures than words. He walks into a Chinatown restaurant with some wild ginseng roots and sits down at a table.

"I just lay them out on the table and wait for someone's eyes to bug out." He wants to surprise people. Given the sight of an old wild ginseng root in the hand of an eccentric-looking white man, he usually doesn't have to wait long.

"Quite often a waiter or waitress will be walking by, and it will catch their eye," he says. "I'll say, 'Bring me dinner and I'll give you these roots.' Next thing you know, they're dragging somebody out of the kitchen. Grandpa, in most cases. And there's a translator, one of the younger ones will translate and say, 'How much do you want for that root?' And I'll say, 'I want you to feed me.' They'll say, 'What?'

"Bring me food," he explains, "not on the menu." Sometimes he brings friends along, too. "And they're just—Oh God, we eat really well."

For three shapely roots, Beyfuss can get a very good dinner. Once he and seven friends were served a six-course seafood dinner, drinks included. It cost him six roots. "I didn't know what the hell I was eating half the time," he says. "I just love Chinese cuisine. It's my favorite cuisine in the whole world."

ONE KEY TO GINSENG's enduring fascination is its story in China, which could be glimpsed in a place Beyfuss has passed many times: the general store at 32 Mott Street, the oldest shop in Manhattan's Chinatown. With its dark shelves crammed with flatware, porcelain, flour, and vegetable seeds, the shop has remained a small antique surrounded by a big new Chinatown. In the late 1800s, it was a neighborhood hub where people bought supplies, paid their bills, and caught up on news from the old country around Fujian. The clerks wrote letters for their customers and read the replies, and on Sundays men gathered for a cup of tea or coffee and swapped stories about family, homes, and business. Until recently, people in the neighborhood still came to 32 Mott Street for news or to pay their wireless phone bill.

There, behind the window display adorned with various herbal soaps (sandalwood, rose, jasmine, and yes, ginseng), are clues to a deeper role that ginseng has played through history. In the back above the long counter hangs an old scale where ginseng and other herbs are measured out. On the wall behind the scale are two strips of wood about three feet long, one dark blue, the other pale yellow. These strips represent imperial banners and illustrate the long arm of the Chinese empire. They used to signal that the shop was a government-authorized retailer of Chinese herbal medicines.

Paul Q. Lee, the shop's owner and a grandson of one of the store's original cofounders, explained. "It's like being the exclusive distributor for Bayer," he told me during one visit. "We were the sole authorized dealer at that time." Besides being the imperial Chinese version of the FDA's seal of approval, the banners show how closely the fortunes of China's emperors were bound to ginseng.

As famous as ginseng is in Chinese medicine, rarely mentioned is the plant's pivotal role in that country's political history, or the fact that one of China's most powerful dynasties was launched by a man who started life as a ginseng trader in a rural horse market.

Power and medicine were never very far apart in ancient China. In the Warring States period (475–221 BC), people who traveled the country's forests and wastelands were urged to carry herbs to protect themselves against deadly diseases like schistosomiasis. Often the medicine served mainly to calm travelers' fears of forces beyond their control, such as wild beasts and flash floods. As time passed and experience sorted out promising plants from the ordinary, ginseng accumulated powerful names throughout China: yellow root, the root that turns its back on the sun, divine herb, the "returned cinnabar with the wrinkled face," and "abounds in spirits." The popular imagination gave ginseng legendary abilities. In one story, a man was repeatedly woken up in the middle of the night by someone calling his name. He would rouse himself and look around, but he never found anyone. One night, at wit's end, he scoured the entire area within a half-mile of his house, and finally stopped before a magnificent ginseng plant that stood as high as his waist. When he dug it out, the root was nearly six feet long and shaped like a man. The cries in the night stopped.

Ginseng could escape from diggers by morphing into a tiger, a man, or a bird. In one Chinese legend, a man happens onto a huge patch of mature ginseng plants. Thrilled, he starts greedily digging them up. Suddenly a little girl appears and starts throwing sand in his eyes. He staggers blindly away, and she chases him so far that he can never find that place again. The girl, of course, was a morphed ginseng plant. The root also was thought to have the power to make itself resemble many other plants, which my ramble with Beyfuss seemed to confirm.

The gist of these stories is that ginseng hunting was never

simply a walk in the woods. To people searching for it, the root acquired the power and cunning of everything in the forest, and finding the plant required courage, discipline, and endurance. Some collectors tried to make themselves worthy of it with strict preparations before the hunt: they abstained from alcohol, meat, and even sex. Running through Chinese manuscripts on the history of ginseng digging is a strong fear that any ginseng plant could suddenly vanish or cause mayhem. As soon as a digger spotted the plant, tradition dictated that he throw himself on the ground and shout, "Don't flee!" He then had to explain quickly that he was a good person and that his motives were pure. If he were with a group expedition, he had to keep shouting until his cries brought others running to help. Then one of them would carefully dig up the root while the first digger kept watch to make sure the plant didn't escape. This notion of a root capable of flight still echoes in stories told by diggers in America.

SUCH A POWERFUL PLANT inevitably drew the attention of the government. Van Symons, a China scholar at Augustana College in Illinois, wrote what may be the only English-language study of ginseng's critical role in China's last dynasty. The Qing dynasty (pronounced "ching") rose to power with a substantial foundation in ginseng money and a monopoly on the ginseng trade.

For centuries, China's emperors struggled unsuccessfully to control how much ginseng people gathered. By the late 1400s, it was nearly extinct in central China, and diggers had moved northward to the land known as Manchuria, and into the Long

White Mountains near Korea. The region was a rough, cold frontier, where emperors exiled their disobedient subjects. Manchuria had rich forests abounding with wildlife and ginseng, and a strange atmosphere that blended gold-rush fever with the air of a penal colony. Its hard-edged native Jurchens (later known as Manchus) ventured only rarely into the Chinese outpost towns inhabited by imperial troops and Han exiles. The Han, China's ethnic majority, regarded the Jurchens as uncouth bumpkins.

In those days, a ginseng digger trekking from the village of Fushun to the regional town of Mukden (present-day Shenyang) would have crossed through a landscape of hardwoods and pine scrub. Mukden was mainly a place to do business with grumpy Han Chinese bureaucrats, but the Jurchen digger would nonetheless encounter some puzzling sights there. The same ginseng and furs that he sold in the market would form part of a much more elaborate spectacle of tribute payments to the emperor. Three times a year, caravans from Korea, a vassal to China, passed through Mukden on their way to Beijing. The envoy from the Korean court and his entourage of forty people or more paraded through with gifts of ginseng and leopard skins (as well as gold, silver, linen, hemp, inlaid boxes, paper, calligraphy brushes, weapons, and slaves). The Korean envoys made money on the side by selling extra roots in Mukden (Korean ginseng sold well). On their return trip they would pass through again, this time loaded up with the emperor's gifts back to the Korean king: jade, robes, musical instruments, medicines, and books—a fantastical display of finery.

One young Jurchen named Nurhaci would eventually grasp the connection between the ginseng roots that he brought to market and the elaborate gifts brought by the rich Korean officials. Nurhaci's grandfather was chief of the Aisin Gioro clan, in the tundra north of the Yalu River. As a teenager in the 1570s, Nurhaci traded ginseng in the Fushun horse market and went with his father on Jurchen tribute missions to Beijing. Although he never learned to read, Nurhaci liked action stories with epic battles and political intrigue, little realizing that his own life would take on those dimensions.

The visits to Beijing piqued his curiosity. Nurhaci was no doubt proud that his family was allied to a powerful general of the Ming court, but his life took a horrific turn when they joined a looting raid that went bad. His grandfather burned to death in a fire set by Ming soldiers, and his father was murdered. Suddenly, the burden of clan leadership landed on Nurhaci's shoulders. He became a target of rivals who provoked him in brawls and sent assassins to his home at night, when he was alone with his family. The Ming court used these rivalries to play one Jurchen faction against another, but in 1586, at age twenty-seven, Nurhaci emerged as the leader. He prospered through two well-connected marriages and ingratiated himself with Beijing, despite its past betrayals. He captured bandits and freed their Chinese hostages. When Japanese aggressors threatened Korea, he offered to lead an army against them. The grateful emperor gave him the title "Dragon-Tiger General."

Nurhaci eventually saw ginseng as a ticket to greater Jurchen power and prestige. He taught Jurchens a new technique for steam-drying the roots that made them softer and more pliant, and therefore easier to transport and more valuable, because they didn't break or rot as easily. He kept a tight focus on the ginseng trade, and as his power grew he sent thousands of men into the Long White Mountains to dig the plant for him. His men apprehended outlaw-ginsenger expeditions and seized their roots as booty.

In time, Nurhaci marshaled enough power to wangle a treaty from Ming generals that gave him control over all ginseng harvests in his territory. His people's profits from the ginseng trade grew to between 30,000 and 90,000 kilograms of silver every year (between $4.5 million and $14.3 million in 2004 dollars). In the summer of 1609, he nearly triggered a war with the Ming court because they were late with payments for ginseng purchases. He sent five thousand troops to collect the money and stopped sending tribute payments to Beijing.

Nurhaci's sense of destiny was crystallizing. He commissioned the creation of a writing system for the Jurchen language and organized his troops with a new system of banners. Grouped under yellow, blue, white, and red flags, his battalions became more efficient and less bound by tribal rivalries. The banners waving overhead became a basis for organizing everything from battle maneuvers to peacetime farming, taxation, and craft-making.

When Nurhaci decided his following was strong enough, he unleashed his pent-up outrage against the Ming rulers. Declaring himself Khan, or emperor, he announced seven grievances against the Ming emperor, including the murders of his father and grandfather. And he complained about how Ming officials mishandled ginseng poachers. Nurhaci led ten thousand troops toward Mukden in a series of stunning victories against a much larger Ming army.

Nurhaci declared Mukden his capital and built a palace that showed his imperial ambitions. Seated on a royal apricot-colored cushion, he dispatched generals and received dignitaries. By the time he died at age sixty-seven, Nurhaci had galvanized his people for a new dynasty in an empire where they had always been outsiders. He had wrestled from Beijing favorable terms for Jurchen ginseng, a trade that fueled their power. As Japanese historian Inaba Iwakichi wrote, "The Qing dynasty rose on ginseng and fell on opium."

Nurhaci's son Huang Taiji built a grand tomb for his father in the wooded hills outside Mukden, carefully situated for good *feng shui* with its back to Tianzhu mountain. (People used the Chinese science of feng shui to channel qi in the landscape just as they used ginseng to direct qi in the body.) The tomb still stands today as a palace for the next world, its great plaza protected by stone animals and watchtowers.

Then Huang Taiji took up his father's ambitions. He dropped the term *Jurchen* and its bumpkin connotations. Instead he called his people *Manchu* and established their dynasty as the Qing. The Chinese characters for Manchu and Qing contain the water symbol, in contrast to the name Ming, which evokes "bright" and "red," and suggests fire. The message was clear: the Qing wave would quench Ming fire. Nurhaci's son launched an assault on Beijing, and although he wouldn't live to see it, the Manchu army breached the Great Wall at Shanhaiguan and marched on the capital in June 1644.

Yet even with their army at Beijing's gates, it was not clear that the Manchus could take power. There again, the economic power of ginseng would be important. As Manchu troops descended on the city, a rival army approached from the south, led by a former postal employee named Li Tzu-ch'eng. Li had led an assembly of bandit groups up and down the Han river basin, and reached the capital weeks before the Manchus. When Li arrived at Beijing, the Ming emperor climbed a hill that commanded a panorama of the Forbidden City and, having lost face, hanged himself.

Now Chinese officials and generals were forced to choose between two invaders: Li or the Manchus. Li notoriously hated the Chinese ruling class. The Manchus were considered barbarians, but posed less of a threat to Chinese culture. They also had the advantage of a strong economic base. So the Manchus were welcomed as the lesser of two evils, and the postman was forced to flee westward after burning the city gates. The Manchus chased him back to the Han valley and nearby mountains, where he was murdered by farmers when he tried to raid their village.

By that autumn, the Manchus held Beijing and were shoring up their economic base. They put the ginseng trade under an imperial monopoly and used Nurhaci's banner system to manage all harvests and sales. The emperor's control over ginseng became even more firm than earlier imperial monopolies over salt. From the customs towers of Beijing's Ch'ungwen Gate, the Ministry of Finance held a taut rein on ginseng that stretched all the way to the Long White Mountains. The Manchus enforced their monopoly with stiff penalties. Any chief who encouraged ginseng poachers was flogged a hundred strokes, a punishment later increased to beheading or strangulation. Tipsters who helped to catch poachers were rewarded with the confiscated property plus up to five ounces of silver for every ounce of root seized.

Once in power, the Manchus tried to protect the forests that had been a source of their power. They set up an epic-scale fence to keep gangs and malcontents out of Manchuria: the "willow palisade" was an embankment planted thick with saplings beside a ditch, intended to serve as a kind of growing Great Wall. Where the Ming had once planted willows to protect Han settlements from Manchu invaders, the Qing emperors turned that idea around: they would guard the Manchu homeland and its forests from Han Chinese intruders from the south. They extended the wall of willow trees for nearly five hundred miles.

Still, the growing Han Chinese population pushed north past the willows and soon was digging ginseng and settling new farms in Manchuria, despite the region's hardships of fierce cold and disease. There were also outlaw gangs, known as blackmen, that poached ginseng from imperial lands, freelance gold miners who staked illegal claims, and other desperate souls who waded icy streams for pearls. (The Chinese had treasured freshwater pearls for over a thousand years; Qing rulers preferred the ones from rivers in their Manchu homeland.)

THE DRAMATIC CHANGES IN China were closely watched by Europe. Through the 1600s, Europeans were hungry for Chinese medicinal herbs such as cinnabar, rhubarb, cassia, camphor, and ginseng. Cinnabar, a crystal form of mercuric sulfide, was used against syphilis and intestinal obstructions. Rhubarb was a common laxative. Cassia bark was valued as a stimulant or antacid, to treat mild diarrhea. Once the English got a toehold in the southern port of Canton, the East India Company's records show, ginseng became one of the main drugs shipped from there, along with rhubarb, cinnabar, and "dragon's blood," a resin used against skin disease (in England it was rumored to be a love charm). A flyer published in London in 1680 described the "root called Nean, or Ninsing," and catalogued its "wonderful Virtue" in curing everything from shortness of breath to "languid tempers." William Simpson, the Yorkshire physician who authored the brochure, had tested a parcel of ginseng and found that it restored an emaciated patient's appetite and ruddy complexion "to the amazement of his desponding relations." In China, Simpson wrote, a pound of ginseng root sold for three times its weight in silver.

The Europeans' only entry point for this valuable trade was the port of Canton, where foreigners had established themselves and Jesuit priests, wearing Chinese clothes and adopting their hosts' customs, had put a sympathetic face on Christianity. By 1651 there were over a hundred thousand Chinese Christians. As the Qing mopped up the last resistance to their rule in the South, they decided not to alienate the missionaries but instead respected the Jesuit accomplishments in science and mapmaking. Nurhaci's great-grandson, the emperor K'ang-hsi (1662–1722), commissioned the Jesuits to make an atlas of his empire. That eight-year mission produced the first map of China to include longitude and latitude. And during the travels for that mission, a French mathematician named Pierre Jartoux made observations about ginseng that would soon bring unexpected consequences a world away, in America.

• • •

Two centuries after Nurhaci sold roots in the horse market and dreamt of power, ginseng diggers were still slogging into Mukden to sell their roots. By the 1700s Mukden had become a greater city, but diggers remained mired in a grim life that shocked foreign visitors. Father Jartoux, for example, was appalled to find ginseng diggers sleeping in the wild without shelter, covered only in branches and leaves. Another traveler found men "wretched in their entire being" who had "no other means of sustaining life than that of giving themselves up, with incredible fatigue, to the search for the ginseng."

A ginseng digger trekked cross-country through "vast and bewildering forests, always left alone to his thoughts and exposed to every discomfort; not knowing if today or tomorrow he may fall victim to the wild beasts that surround him."

"Our work is difficult and dangerous," one digger told another foreigner in the 1800s. The task was grueling emotionally as well as physically, since diggers were sure that their quarry had supernatural powers. Before finding the ginseng, diggers had to fight off its henchmen: the root was often reportedly guarded by panthers and a big tiger she-cat. (The digger quoted above said that in six years of pursuing ginseng he had killed nine tigers, two panthers, and several bears.) Even more terrifying was the little devil with glowing red eyes who would set the underbrush on fire to flush diggers away. "It also happens that the devil takes the form of the ginseng root," that digger added. "When the hunter approaches it, the root retreats further and further, until the man loses his way and perishes in the forest."

A digger had to set out into the hills even before the winter had ended and the spring thaw made the northern rivers treacherous. He loaded provisions onto a snow sledge and set out early, or else had to canoe or pack into the wilderness and risk losing the best claims. A digger would plan to spend the spring and summer out in the wild, but the government limited his supplies to keep him from provisioning outlaws. He could take just six pecks of grain, and a pack animal only if it had a government brand. He was also barred from taking seeds or spears or hunting dogs. The government only wanted diggers out there to get ginseng, not to make a life for themselves. And all along the way, they got short-changed. One year officials siphoned off up to 80 percent of the money designated for ginseng diggers.

Diggers were taken to designated ginseng concession areas by military escort, and had to return under escort, too, according to a schedule. Once encamped in the forest, a ginseng digger would set out in the morning with a small knife, a bag of tinder, a digging stick (he could only use tools made of wood or bone, to prevent scratching the precious roots) and a leather bag for roots. He crawled through thickets wearing a coarse blue shirt and trousers, moccasins, a birchbark hat, and a leather apron to keep from getting dew-soaked and stung by nettles. At the end of the day he trudged back to camp and spent the evening washing, scraping, and boiling his roots with the same technique Nurhaci had used—often steaming his dinner in a double-boiler at the same time. Finally he would string the roots on a line to dry, eat his dinner, and prepare for another day.

The palace set impossibly high ginseng quotas. The Manchu homeland grew more lawless, and the Qing emperors lost control of ginseng harvests. More and more they were losing control of China itself. The Imperial Household realized it couldn't stop poachers, it could only compete with them. As China scholar Van Symons explained to me, officials hungry for revenues set the quotas knowing that poachers would get any roots that licensed diggers left behind. Public demand was soaring, stoked by merchants who exaggerated ginseng's healing abilities. Charlatans claimed it could revive the dying. Ginseng carried the ultimate status: long life and official power. Europeans commented on the high ceremony that surrounded the plant. William Lockhart, a missionary doctor in Shanghai in the 1840s, visited a ginseng merchant and was struck by the elaborate ritual that his host used to unveil the root from fine silks, and the accompanying tea ceremony.

Resigned that ginseng would be overharvested no matter what, the imperial court decided to reap the plant's riches while it could. Diggers were sent deeper into the hills and endured more hardships; roots became still harder to find. In the end, China's last dynasty ebbed and the wild root vanished from its forests.

FOUR

Life in a New World

*In China, Your Grace, there is not a single plant
that can compare to Ginseng.*

—FATHER JOSEPH-FRANÇOIS LAFITAU,
scholar-missionary, Paris, 1718

AUTUMN IS STILL THE season for wild ginseng, but these
days more of it passes through lower Manhattan than
through Mukden. Wild American ginseng, specifically, accumu-
lates in the storerooms of a few wholesale exporters in New York
(as well as San Francisco and Seattle), before getting weighed
and shipped to Asia.

Mid-September finds David Law, America's largest exporter
of wild ginseng, seated in his Manhattan office five minutes
north of Chinatown, pondering his next steps. Law is debating,
as he says, "when to get the engine started." This involves complex calculations. Are diggers demanding too high a price early
in the season? Will it go down? It's like the stock market, Law
says; you don't want to jump into buying ginseng at the wrong
time or you'll take a bath. The right time is usually around the
twentieth of September. That's when the engine starts.

"Whether or not I make a living depends on two months: mid-September to mid-November." David Law speaks in quick, energetic bursts. When he talks about ginseng, his voice goes down and then swoops high, punctuated by occasional spurts of laughter.

"This year I think I'll stay off a little bit," he tells me. "I think the price will get as high as possible." Bob Beyfuss, too, mentioned that ginseng's price was high that season. Starting from about $100 per pound of fresh roots, buyers were suddenly paying twice that. (The price for fresh roots is usually a good deal less than for dried roots, since drying concentrates the valuable root matter. The Chinese market prefers dried ginseng, but in Korea consumers pay a premium for fresh roots.) "There's one buyer who seems to be driving up the price," Beyfuss had said. "I don't know who's bankrolling him." This would become a theme throughout that fall: everybody knew the price for wild ginseng was up; nobody seemed to know what was causing it.

GINSENG'S LIFE IN THE New World was fraught with nearly as much power and peril as it was in China. Empires rose and fell. Plants appeared and disappeared. The story of how the hunt for wild ginseng was relocated from Asia to America led me from Law's office up the Hudson to the Mohawk River. About the time when Nurhaci's followers were storming Beijing, Europeans were charging up the Mohawk Valley to the League of the Iroquois, a group of five nations that Hiawatha united in the late 1400s. (Besides the Mohawk, the league included the Oneidas, Onondagas, Cayugas, and Senecas.) If money from furs and ginseng together was what propelled the

Manchus to power in China, Europeans were drawn to America mainly by the desire for furs. They simply didn't know ginseng from poison ivy. But the Iroquois did; colonial observers in the mid 1700s noted the use of American ginseng among many Native American groups. The Penobscots in Maine reportedly took ginseng to improve fertility, and the Menominee in Wisconsin used it as a tonic that improved mental sharpness. The Micmac employed ginseng as a "detergent for the blood." Down at the southern end of the Appalachian chain, where Tennessee met North Carolina, the Cherokee used ginseng against convulsions, palsy, vertigo, dysentery, headache, colic, and thrush.

There's debate, however, about whether Native Americans used ginseng extensively before it became valuable in trade with China. Steven Archer, an anthropologist at Berkeley, doubts that ginseng played a large role in the lives of Native Americans. Archer has studied archaeological remains at farm sites in colonial Virginia dating to the late 1600s, searching for clues to indigenous knowledge that passed from Algonquin residents to Europeans. Ginseng, he told me, "may not have been a big deal before European contact." Colonial Virginians learned many health lessons from the Algonquins, from snakebite remedies to sassafras, but Archer found no sign of ginseng. "My hunch is that the commercial value of ginseng was probably the key factor in incorporating it into the Native American pharmacopoeia," he added. Bob Beyfuss was equally unconvinced that ginseng was widely used by Native Americans before the China trade. "That's another big argument I had with the people at the New York Encyclopedia," he told me. "I mean, Native Americans knew the plant—they knew all the plants. And they used it—they used all the plants. But I don't think it was an important medicine."

This was a disagreement I couldn't resolve. In following the root and its history, I was reminded of a line from Lao Tze on the distinction between the path that can be named and the path that cannot. In the world of people I found almost too many words about ginseng. But on the plant's home turf in the forest, the competing words gave way to silence and a life lived far from any language. Legends about roots that screamed in the night or that fled further into the forest, were, I figured, attempts to express things that happened in the wordless realm of nature—fears, frustrations, and desires.

Soon after my visit with Beyfuss, I drove to a Mohawk community near Fonda, west of Albany, hoping to find out how Native American groups actually used ginseng. The community held workshops on Iroquois herbology and healing, where a prominent Iroquois herbalist had shown people how to pick, dry, and prepare medicinal herbs. Last time the herbalist and her students had found over forty types of medicinal plants in the woods.

As I drove west on I-90, stone bluffs rose up on the river's south bank. I left the highway and soon several signs flashed past me, announcing the Mohawk Bed and Breakfast and the Mohawk Craft Shop.

"You are in the valley of the Bear Clan of the Mohawk," said the woman behind the counter in the craft shop of Kanatsio-hareke (gah-nah-JO-hah-LA-gay). The name is the Mohawk word for "clean pot" and comes from the stone pockets in the nearby limestone creek. She explained that for two centuries after they were chased from this valley, the Mohawk nurtured a dream that someday they would return. Finally in 1993 a Mohawk leader named Tom Porter had enough support to buy ninety acres of farmland here. He turned three old wood frame buildings into a latter-day longhouse and named the place Kanatsiohareke. At the time of my visit fourteen people lived there, practicing a more-or-less traditional Mohawk lifestyle except for e-mail and a few other technologies that didn't conflict with those traditions. The medicinal plant weekend was one of several workshops designed to reinvigorate those same Mohawk (and more broadly, Iroquois) traditions.

This area was the first home of the Mohawks who later showed ginseng to the Jesuit missionary who documented it for the world. Mary, the craft-shop manager, had come to Kanatsiohareke six years earlier from New York City, where she had grown up and worked for years as a film editor. She was proud of the Iroquois knowledge of plants and equally conversant on global climate change. We talked for over an hour, and I learned about participatory Iroquois government and politics. She sold me a copy of the Mohawk Thanksgiving Address.

By the time I stepped outside, the sun was low to my right, and across the river the steep, conifer-covered bluffs known as Big Nose and Little Nose had turned a warm ochre. At the left edge of the farm property, a stream bed was blooming with purple lythrum. That was the shallow stream with the limestone pockets that gave this place its name. Here was the site of a Mohawk village where a Dutch merchant and Indian trader named LaJelles Fonda had made his home, according to a historical marker by the road. Fonda's great-grandfather, a Dutch whaler, had come to the valley in the 1640s when it was a hotspot in the European trade war over furs. The Mohawk River valley was the gateway into the League of the Iroquois, which stretched westward to Lake Erie, and influenced life as far west as the Mississippi River. For thousands of years the Mohawk valley had given the Iroquois a path to the coast. The Dutch traders were coming in the other direction, followed by the French and the English.

European visitors saw in this landscape idyllic versions of their own memories—mountains "so exceedingly high that they appear to almost touch the clouds," one wrote, pausing to admire the fir trees, oaks, alders, chestnuts, elms, plums, walnuts, blueberries, strawberries, and wild grape. Waterfowl filled the skies (swans, geese, widgeons, teal, brant, and ducks) and fish of all kinds teemed in the "excellent river"—catfish, pike, perch, lampreys, eels, sunfish, bass, and shad. In the spring, a man with a hook and line could catch more perch in an hour than a dozen men could eat.

Some travelers commented on Mohawk life and health care. In the 1630s a Dutchman named Harmen van den Bogaert was traveling up the valley with two other fur traders and found villages reeling from a smallpox epidemic that followed an earlier wave of Dutch travelers, killing half the population. Van den Bogaert reported everything from the pungent smell of dried salmon to the Mohawks' hospitality and their meals of baked boiled pumpkins, beans, and venison. He was a barber-surgeon, performing operations along the way ("I made some cuts with a knife in Willem Tomssen's leg," went one entry, "and then smeared it with bear's grease") and taking notes on local medical practices. When Mohawk doctors built a large fire to sweat out a patient's illness, Van den Bogaert watched as they soaked medicines in water, stuck them down their own throats, and then vomited on the patient's head. Other Europeans were more impressed by the Mohawk combination of a sauna and a leap into a cold stream, and by their "wonderful" treatment of wounds and injuries using "herbs, roots, and leaves from the land." Women were the ones who gathered the medicinal roots, along with firewood and wild nuts, berries, greens, and mushrooms. (They also did the farming, made clothing, cooked the food, made maple sugar in the spring.) The men cleared the fields for crops and went on hunting expeditions.

On the opposite shore from where I stood, beneath the bluffs that looked warm and glowing at sunset, the French came in the autumn of 1666 and destroyed Mohawk villages and crops in order to secure their access to the fur trade. Eventually the Mohawk made up with the French and allowed Jesuit missionaries into their village of Caughnawaga. When the English muscled into the valley, the Jesuits and their Mohawk converts were sent packing northward to Montreal. The villagers took along their possessions, including their ginseng.

Mohawk and other Iroquois used ginseng and other wild plants in medicine primarily to give thanks and practice preventive health care. In *Iroquois Medical Botany,* a botanical compendium by anthropologist James Herrick, American ginseng is listed as a remedy for sore eyes (boil a small root in a cup of water, squeeze drops into eyes every hour), tapeworms, vomiting, bad appetite, earaches, and a difficult childbirth. For an upset stomach, boil roots in a quart of water. "Drink all you can," urged the text.

For the Iroquois, everything and everyone possessed a life force, or *orenda,* which could influence other parts of the cosmos. In Iroquois culture, "the key unifying principle was that of harmony or balance," and so they tried to balance orenda through repeated greetings and thank-yous to nature. But before I could try to connect the dots between Iroquois and Taoist philosophies and their search for balance, Herrick insisted that instead of puzzling over why traditional societies share these broad views, we might ask why the Western world view *doesn't* share a belief in balance. Why does Western thought prefer to break things down into small, separate categories?

For the Iroquois, too, everything had a purpose from the Creator. Every plant had its use, and it was the duty of people to remind it of that use. A speech of thanksgiving performed that function and created a bond between the person who spoke it and the plant.

The Iroquois Thanksgiving Address offered a clue to how significant the Iroquois considered an item like ginseng, Herrick suggested. Things with narrower uses usually got thanked early in the address, and items with more universal functions came later. I found medicinal herbs thanked halfway through, after food plants and before all animal life. Medicinal herbs, the address said, "are always waiting and ready to heal us. We are happy there are still among us those special few [people] who remember how to use these plants for healing. With one mind, we send greetings and thanks to the Medicines and to the keepers of the Medicines."

The Iroquois viewed the body's tendency to heal as proof that nature leans toward balance: a scab forms over a wound and falls off, revealing new whole skin. Modern Americans often see traditional medicine either negatively, as an unscientific novelty, or through a romantic lens, as an exotic set of long-lost secrets to the universe. Herrick considered the mechanisms of traditional medicine to be more straightforward. One "secret" that Westerners often forget is the need to reduce stress and allow the body's healing properties to work, Herrick wrote. Faith in any kind of medicine reduces stress. Regardless of what medical system you follow, the attitude "Medicine helps" contributes at least a little to healing because it helps us relax. Freed from stress, the body can devote itself to healing. This falls in the realm of the placebo effect but is different from the delusion usually implied by that term. Herrick suggested that when medical researchers dismiss the placebo effect as background noise, they dismiss a mechanism that helps any medicine work. In scientific terms, however, it's not reproducible, and Western science relies on replicable results in its progress toward truth.

GINSENG IN THE AMERICAS was not just used in medicine. It was part of the landscape of the mountains, from the Iroquois league south to the Cherokee. So I visited the town of Cherokee, North Carolina, during the ninetieth annual Cherokee Indian Fair. At night people parked beside my motel and walked to the fairground where the amusement rides glowed with fluorescent lights. They were all ages, like visitors to any county fair. I followed them past food tents and a row of vendors selling frybread, burgers, and Indian dinners (beanbread, greens, beans and hominy, chicken and fatback). On the green, eight-year-olds tackled each other and compared shoes. The eight finalists in the Teen Miss Cherokee Pageant waved, sang, walked the catwalk, and performed dances and chants. One contestant recited a poem, "To a U.S. Warrior," that blended the war on terror with tribal metaphors. The evening closed with an Elvis impersonator rocking through "Johnny B. Goode" and "Suspicious Minds."

The Eastern band of the Cherokee traces its history back to a people known for the great earthworks they made in the hills of what is now western North Carolina. In the 1790s, the Quaker naturalist William Bartram noted the Cherokee reverence for ginseng in his *Travels,* which became a bestselling adventure memoir. The Cherokee spoke of the plant as a sentient being, Bartram wrote, "able to make itself invisible to those unworthy to gather it." Being worthy meant not being greedy: taking just one plant in four, and repaying any harvested root with a bead, a prayer, and a replacement seed. It meant giving thanks.

In the winter of 1838, the U.S. government used a fraudulent treaty to force the Cherokee from their ancestral lands throughout the Southeast. As a result fifteen thousand Cherokee were marched nearly a thousand miles, west of the Mississippi, on a trek that became known as the Trail of Tears. Nearly a third of them died on the way. Left behind in the hills of North Carolina was a small group of Cherokee known as the Oconaluftee. The Oconaluftee had separated from other Cherokees almost twenty years before, saying that the Cherokee Nation's efforts to modernize marked a betrayal of their traditions. Ironically, the more traditional Oconaluftee were allowed to stay in North Carolina because they weren't bound by the bad treaty, while the modernizing Cherokees were forced westward. Along with a few who escaped the march, the Oconaluftee remained in their mountains and through the 1800s sold ginseng to white traders for shipment to China. Historian Barbara Duncan writes that proceeds from ginseng sales probably helped the Eastern Cherokee buy back more of their ancestral lands. They have continued to collect and sell ginseng through to the present.

A century ago medicine shows traveled these hills. There were white medicine shows and black medicine shows, and some that combined Cherokee herbalism with the African tradition of root-doctoring. Ginseng was a regular headliner in Lotus Flower Medicine and other cures. Not far from the town of Cherokee, Phoebe Sullivan, who described herself as part white, part black, and part Cherokee, dispensed herbal medicine and Christian teachings for decades, until she died in 1960. Patients came from as far as Detroit for appointments with her and for her medicines, including yellowroot and ginseng, which she paid herb gatherers to collect.

I strolled through the Cherokee fair with an eye peeled for ginseng. One tent held displays of prize-winning crafts and foods—canned beans and a blue-ribbon pumpkin two feet in diameter, delicious-looking peach and pumpkin pies—but no old-time medicinal herbs.

The next day at the Museum of the Cherokee, tribe elder Jerry Wolf agreed to talk with me about ginseng after he finished his lunch. Wolf worked at the museum several days a week and kept himself involved in Cherokee ceremonies like one that dedicated a trail at the Sequoyah Birthplace Museum in Vonore, Tennessee. While waiting, I walked through the museum's permanent exhibit, pausing at the Mississippi Era diorama of a little hogan. Suddenly a holographic shaman stepped out and tossed some grains onto a holographic bonfire. It flared brightly and gave off smoke with a crackling sound.

"That's powerful medicine," the shaman said. Then he told the Cherokee story of how disease originated. It said that animals inflicted illness on man as their revenge on hunters. Medicine came about when the plants of the world took pity on humans and offered them a remedy for most diseases. As a result of the plants' generosity, there's a cure for every disease that the animals inflicted, and every plant has a use, if we know what it is. (On that point the Cherokee agreed with the Iroquois.) The little holographic shaman then exited.

Jerry Wolf came downstairs and we went outside and sat on a stone bench. The museum stood next to the Cherokee fairgrounds, so as we talked people stopped to say hello to Wolf or ask a question. He always answered patiently. Two huge young museum staffers who had been working in the gift shop hailed him on their way to the parking lot, headed for lunch. One had a tattoo on his close-cropped scalp.

"They need to eat, don't they?" Wolf said after they passed. "They're starving to death."

His voice was a gentle baritone like the actor Dennis Weaver's. Wolf was slender and wore a pale shirt with the museum's logo, a beaded tie, and a black, wide-brimmed hat with a Stars and Stripes sticker on the back. At seventy-seven, Wolf was beginning to stoop but was still light on his feet. On his right forearm were two tattoos: one of a young Indian woman's face and one representing his unit in the Navy.

Wolf knew ginseng well, mainly from the perspective of

someone who collects it in the woods. He had hunted ginseng since selling his first roots to country stores when he was growing up, in the 1930s and 1940s. He recalled people trading roots for groceries. With the museum at our backs, Wolf shifted into Cherokee legends and storytelling. "We have a name for it in the Cherokee language," he said. *"Ah-dili-gah-lee. Ah-dili-gah-lee."* The word had its own rolling rhythm that contrasted with the plant's staccato English name (which was itself a corruption of its Cantonese name).

Wolf said the mountains, too, sounded completely different in Cherokee. "There's a good example right through there." He pointed at a sharp, coned summit to the north. "Right below those clouds heaping up there. That's called Rattlesnake Mountain. Rattlesnake Mountain," he repeated. "I don't know how they got that name, but that's the English name for it. The Cherokee name is *Atsilawo-i. Atsilawo-i* means 'covered with fire.' See the difference?"

The mountain's Cherokee name came from the story of a great snake with a crystal on its head that drew prey like a magnet. The snake's body was as thick as a tree trunk and covered with glittering scales. (One scholar has noticed a "marked similarity" between the snake-with-the-crystal-on-its-head legend and the dragon of Chinese mythology.) Wolf said that like the crystal, the mountain would light up every so often. One night his son looked up at the mountain and saw a big ball of fire up on its summit.

Ginseng, by contrast, had the power to repel people, especially those who look for it. To defuse that power, the Cherokee traditionally had a shaman call on a spirit to help them find ginseng. Sometimes the shaman would give the ginseng seeker a chant and tell him to go toward something fearful, for example a bear or a snake, in order to find the plant. Wolf told a story from his own experience. "I was back in the mountains," he said, "and I came back to a big rock cliff. There was a rock that you could sit on, just like this." He patted our stone bench.

"I was ginseng-digging and I came to this and I sat down," he said. "And I started breaking out my sandwich." Then, on a moment's inspiration, he broke off a piece of the sandwich and tossed it in the crevice at the base of the cliff and said in Cherokee, "Help me find what I'm looking for."

"I said, '*Eks deya sadong hey honga du si.*' I said it like that. Well, I started eating my sandwich. It wasn't long before I heard a noise back in there. And I thought, 'My gosh, is that real? Is that noise coming from in the crevice?' And then I'd look around and I'd stick my head out and listen."

Wolf told himself to finish his sandwich and not get scared. "I got up. I went around this big rock—you had to go around quite a ways. About from here to that wall." He gestured to a spot about twenty feet away. "And it was *rough* in that area. Straight up and down, like these mountains. Just *straight* up and down. And I got around that rock cliff and I looked down the way I had come, and I saw a *big* ginseng, standing there like this."

Wolf put his hand out about thirty inches off the ground.

"Do you know, just in that little area, I found a big bunch of ginseng? And it was time for the berries, too, so I sowed all the berries back." He added, "Somebody told me it was probably the little people, back in there. There's a lot of different tribes of little people in these Great Smokies."

The Cherokee knew the local flora so well that they could go fishing without either hook or spear, using only poisonous plants like devil's shoestring or goat's rue *(Tephrosia virginiana)* and red buckeye *(Aesculus pavia)* that, when immersed in small pools, would paralyze fish without rendering them inedible.

In the Cherokee sacred formulas, ginseng was addressed by a name that translates as "Little Person" or "little man of the mountain." According to Cherokee medicine man Hawk LittleJohn, ginseng was a symbol of balance and harmony. "You take it in the winter and it strengthens you like sunlight," LittleJohn told an interviewer. (Their version of balance was not entirely peaceful. In Cherokee justice, balance meant an eye for an eye. One life balanced another: a murdered person's family could restore balance only by killing the murderer. Any Cherokee who left such an imbalance unaddressed forfeited his own right to live. "If men neglected to avenge the deaths of their kinsmen," wrote local historian Theda Perdue, "others would be free to kill them without fear, as men are free to kill bears.")

Jerry Wolf seemed far removed from the Cherokee sacred formulas, but he still respected ginseng's powers and the need to repay the plant for its harvest. He taught his children how to recognize the plant in the wild, too, even though they showed no interest in digging it.

"It's a strange plant," Wolf said. "If you find a big patch of ginseng, it's usually just about dark. It's too late to dig it. You're in a hurry to get back to your car, or walk home, or wherever you are. And you can mark it or do anything you want to find that area, and think, 'I'll be back tomorrow and dig it.' You go back tomorrow, you'll never find that place. Never. You won't find it.

"You better dig it right then." Wolf explained why with a story of a knife he lost.

He was up in the mountains looking for ginseng. "I remember cutting some briars. And there was a ginseng mixed in with all those briars, so we had to cut the briars out to get into where you could dig the 'sang without getting scratched up. And I got back in. I took my knife out, cut them all, got it clear. But when I found the ginseng standing there, I looked over here and I looked over there, to see if there was any more. There was no other 'sang anywhere. I got down and dug it. Meantime I lost the knife.

"I got home that night, and I told my wife, I said, 'I lost my knife in the woods.' And I said, 'That's an expensive knife. I'm going back in the morning and I'm going to see if I can find it.'

"I got back up to the area after a hard, long hike. I finally found the place where I had been. I wasn't really looking for ginseng. I was looking for my knife, because that was the last place I used it that I could remember. And I looked around and I didn't see the knife. But not far from where I had dug that big one was another one this tall." Wolf raised his open palm two feet off the ground. "I pointed my finger at that ginseng and I said, 'You weren't there yesterday. You were not there yesterday!'

"It's a *strange* plant," he stressed. "It will be there and it won't."

MEANDERING CONVERSATIONS ABOUT strange plants could yield astonishing results and had, in fact, led directly to

the multimillion-dollar trade in American ginseng. Such was
the experience of Father Lafitau, the man who uncovered the
link between American and Asian ginseng.

Joseph-François Lafitau, an eighteenth-century Jesuit cleric,
made a discovery near Montreal that set in motion the reunion
of yin and yang roots, and launched American ginseng's travels
around the globe. Although little known today, Father Lafitau's
name is recognized almost like a password among longtime
ginsengers and root traders. He was born in Bordeaux, France,
on New Year's Day, 1681, into a family of bankers and wine merchants. (At that time in China, Nurhaci's dynasty was less than
forty years old.) Bordeaux was a major Atlantic port, and had a
long history with vineyards and trade. The city prospered on a
triangular commerce: slaves from Africa went to the French
West Indies; coffee and sugar from the Indies went to Bordeaux;
and wine and guns left Bordeaux for Africa. In the harbor young
Lafitau saw ships from the Antilles, New France (that is, Canada),
and South America. Sailors and traders filled the streets with
foreign languages, and city festivals displayed Native Americans
as exhibits.

Lafitau absorbed these sights and sounds. Always bookish,
he joined the Jesuits while still a teenager, studied philosophy
and rhetoric, and then taught grammar in the mountainous
Massif Central region. He eventually finished his theology
studies in Paris. At that point the Enlightenment was dawning.
Scholars were expected to go beyond theory and draw conclu-
sions from observing the world. The Jesuits were well suited to
meet that challenge, since they combined scholarship with energetic missionary work abroad. They were closely allied with

the pope and had a strong political arm that often involved them in diplomacy.

On April 10, 1711, Lafitau petitioned his father superior for permission to go work as a missionary among the Iroquois. It wasn't clear why he wanted to. He wasn't a parish priest or a naturalist intrigued by a new land. Lafitau was more at home in the world of ideas. He was uninterested in landscapes, or as William Fenton, an Iroquois scholar, later put it, "unaware of the beauties of silent rivers and deep forests of the New World." Permission was granted — Lafitau would set sail at the end of the year. He spent the summer and fall of 1711 in his hometown, teaching rhetoric to college students and preparing for the journey.

LAFITAU REACHED QUEBEC in the early, icy months of 1712 and immediately went upriver to Montreal to immerse himself in the world of the Iroquois. His first task was to learn their language from missionaries who had spent decades brokering treaties among the North American tribes. He learned most from Father Julien Garnier, an energetic veteran of nearly half a century on the western frontier who had spent his entire adulthood among the Iroquois. Lafitau later paid tribute to Garnier as a mentor of rare "understanding and knowledge." With Garnier as his first guide, Lafitau plunged into everything about the Iroquois: how they prepared food, how they cleared the fields, how the women tended the crops. He listened and quoted them at length in his journal, even their defenses of customs that, as a missionary, he was supposed to discourage. He reports one Mohawk woman's protests when he urged her to stop using a divining fire to predict events:

I have never understood what harm there is in it and I still have great difficulty in seeing any. Listen, God has given men different gifts. To the Frenchmen, he has given the Scriptures by which you learn the things which take place far from you as if they were in front of you; to us he has given the art of knowing, by fire, things remote in time or place. Suppose then that this fire is our book, our Scriptures, thou willst not see that there is any difference or more harm in the one than in the other. My mother taught me this secret in my infancy as thy parents taught thee to read and write. I used it successfully several times before I became a Christian. I have done it sometimes with some success since. I have been tempted and yielded to temptation but without thinking that I was committing any sin.

He may even have been secretly delighted by her comparison of her divining fire with his own books. Such observations were drawing him toward knowledge that the Mohawk rarely shared, including their use of ginseng.

He was assigned to a settlement called Sault St. Louis, known in Iroquois as Caughnawaga. Opposite Montreal on the south bank of the St. Lawrence, the village was home to the six hundred Mohawk converts who had been uprooted from a village of the same name two hundred miles south, on the Mohawk River near Tom Porter's present-day settlement of Kanatsiohareke. Using their knowledge of the terrain between British Albany and French Montreal, the villagers plied a dangerous but profitable contraband business while England and France battled for the fur trade.

The scholar-priest was intrigued not just by their outer life, but also by the Iroquois view of dreams; he wrote about how they felt their lives depended on granting wishes expressed in dreams. Certain dreams obligated the dreamer and the community to fulfill them or else everyone risked terrible consequences. Such a belief obviously opened possibilities for corruption. Lafitau recounts a battle of wills that followed after an Iroquois man met a French trapper with a nice blanket. The Iroquois asked for the blanket, and since he had dreamt of owning it, the trapper granted the request. Within days, though, the trapper said he had dreamt of the Iroquois' fine buffalo robe; the owner handed it over.

> These alternating daydreams went on for some time, the Indian continuing to dream and the Frenchman having always a return dream. . . . Finally the Indian grew tired first. He went to find the Frenchman and made him agree that they would no longer dream of one another's possessions.

Lafitau's commentaries often suggest more sympathy for pagan beliefs than a missionary could safely admit. In his description of the Iroquois marriage ritual, you can almost hear him burble an apology to the church censor: "It appears of the simplest nature but I can say that it is all sacramental, so to speak, if I dare express myself thus. . . ." Lafitau always considered an item from several angles. He admired the craftsmanship of Iroquois canoes, for example, yet complained they were awkward and their elm bark construction wasn't as good as the Algonquins' birch bark canoes.

In October 1715 Lafitau was visiting the Jesuit mission in

Quebec and saw, in their copy of the order's newsletter from France, an item that caught his attention. An article by Father Pierre Jartoux, the Jesuit mathematician who had traveled through Mongolia to make an atlas of China, described Asian ginseng and its value in Chinese medicine. Dated 1713, Jartoux's article told of meeting with ten thousand people sent to collect ginseng for the emperor, and how his hosts in China had given him four ginseng plants to try. Jartoux wrote that, after an hour, "I found my Pulse much fuller and quicker, I had an Appetite, and found myself much more vigorous." He tried the root again four days later, when he was so exhausted he could hardly stay in the saddle. An hour later he felt good as new. Jartoux reported that ginseng lived up to its Chinese reputation as a restorative, and described the plant's botany, preparation, and mountainous habitat. Almost as an afterthought, he added that it might possibly grow in a similar environment in the New World.

The article intrigued Lafitau. He became fixated on it, in fact, and quietly dedicated himself to finding a plant in the Canadian wilderness for which he had no name, with barely any reason to think that it might grow there. Winter passed, and finally spring came and flushed. Although careful not to draw attention to his efforts or risk being seen as condoning pagan beliefs, Lafitau took time from his mission work to search for the plant, and asked Mohawk herbalists and others about the plants they used. He made field trips into the forest, and described again and again what he was looking for to his Mohawk sources, as well as to Huron and Abenaqui. His intensity proved contagious, and soon they wanted to find the plant as much as he did.

After three months of searching and puzzling, he finally found a plant that matched Jartoux's description of the Chinese panacea, right near a house he was having built. It was a mature plant "whose vermillion fruit captured my attention." Lafitau couldn't believe it might really be the plant he had been searching for. Wracked with eagerness, he carried it to a Mohawk woman he had hired to help him. Sure, she said, she knew that little bush. It was one of their common cures; her people used it for minor complaints, but not with the same fervor as the newsletter indicated in China. Lafitau urged the woman (whom he didn't name) to boil the crushed root the way that Jartoux described, and drink the decoction. She did, and it cured an intermittent fever that had bothered her for months.

To confirm his hopes, he sent for the copy of the newsletter article and botanical illustrations he had seen in Quebec. When that arrived, he brought some fresh roots into his cabin and compared them with the engravings. Lafitau's Mohawk advisors confirmed that they were the same plant. Holding them side by side, he wrote later, "we had the pleasure of seeing a description so exact . . . that it did not lack the least detail of which we had the proof before our eyes."

This reunion of American ginseng with its Asian cousin was by no means inevitable. There are surely dozens of species of hydrangeas and magnolias that have never reconnected with their relatives across the Pacific. Most of the two continents' shared history remains unexplored. It was the agency of human enterprise—human desires for health, or wealth, or power— that would carry wild American ginseng roots halfway around the world, to be sold in Canton beside Asian roots. But in another sense it wasn't human enterprise alone; the wild root's own shape and interaction with the human body helped to enlist people to make the voyage happen. For the Iroquois, words of thanksgiving confirmed a bond between a plant and the person who knew its use. Jartoux's newsletter article about ginseng in China offered something almost as sacred for Father Lafitau: an idea.

By then, Lafitau had spent three years with the Iroquois and was starting to see parallels between their ways of life and customs he had read about in the literature of ancient Greece and Rome. He was always looking for connections and parallels, and Jartoux's article had piqued his curiosity because he suspected that the Chinese use of ginseng might correspond with some of the remarkable Iroquois remedies. Ultimately, as it has done for so many others, ginseng supplied Lafitau with a focus for his passions. Lafitau reasoned that if the Chinese plant ginseng really did grow in both the New World and the Orient, the plant might be an outward and visible sign of a hidden and ancient connection between the two worlds. If Lafitau could find evidence that linked how America's natives used plants with the ways the Chinese used them, he would have a foundation for arguing that American Indians originally came from the Old World.

Furthermore, there might be worldly benefits to finding ginseng. Jesuits in South America had had great success discovering useful plants. Lafitau felt that his colleagues were missing equally important opportunities in Canada simply because they disregarded the knowledge of the people there. Lafitau understood that progress for Christianity and the Jesuits was tightly woven with the progress of France. From his upbringing in Bordeaux and his training as a Jesuit, an order that approached its mission with an entrepreneurial eye, Lafitau would have anticipated the French government's desire to extract a valuable resource from Canada.

His main interest, though, was larger than commerce. Lafitau's use of Jartoux's illustrations became the first documented use of botanical drawings in field research, and his research method made him a father of comparative anthropology. The *Encyclopedia Britannica* counts him among the four most important chroniclers of non-European religions of his age.

Within months of his discovery, however, Lafitau was called back to Paris and became caught up in litigation over the sale of liquor to Indians. The son of wine merchants had to testify for a ban against liquor sales in the colonies.

In Paris, Lafitau found himself surrounded by a society at odds with his beliefs, and a jarring contrast from the Iroquois world where he had spent the last five years. The Iroquois priorities were survival and loyalty; Paris was obsessed with luxury. Lafitau could barely restrain his contempt. He countered rumors of American promiscuity by pointing out that in Europe "we see, everywhere, unbridled license and boundless scandal which would horrify the Indians themselves." He contrasted the hardy Iroquois with the "soft, lazy life" of Europeans and their "excess and variety of wines."

Lafitau completed the account of his discovery of ginseng in America thirty years after the Sun King had celebrated his first gift of Asian ginseng at Versailles. A Paris publisher on the

narrow Rue St. Jacques put it out as a booklet addressed to the
Duke of Orleans, the crown regent and patron of the Jesuits.

Today Lafitau's book is as elusive as the plant it describes. After many hours spent in musty library stacks, it was a thrill for me
to come across an original edition. In the shell of translucent marble that holds Yale's rare book collection, a librarian brought out
the slim volume bound in red-and-gilt leather, not much larger
than a three-by-five index card. On the spine it said simply,

Lafitau
La Plante
du
Gin-Seng

Inside, an intricate centerfold of botanical drawings depicted
a four-prong plant with berries and root. The centerfold also included drawings of not one but five different roots, over a dozen
wrinkles on each neck, a cross-sectional view, and flowers and
bracts. (Typically, the restless Lafitau critiqued even these illustrations: "badly done," he grumbled in the text, citing another
book where the images were better.)

Lafitau, always the exhaustive researcher, began his account
with a survey of the literature, building a case from Jartoux and
other sources, documenting ginseng's use and fame in China.
The miracle herb restored lost energy. It grew on black, granu-
lar soils and preferred shade. It cost a fortune. Then he recounted the detective story of his research: the months of
searching for the plant in Canada, the help of the Iroquois
woman, and the confirmation, using Jartoux's engravings, that
Asian ginseng and American ginseng were virtually identical.

Same plant, two continents. He added that the plant's Iroquois name, *Garent-oguen,* translated as very similar to the Chinese name: "resembles man." The discovery held great promise, since the plant was abundant in Canada.

Lafitau's booklet ignited an excitement comparable to what the California Gold Rush inspired a century later. The timing was perfect: Louis XIV's gift of Asian ginseng roots from the Siamese ambassador had spurred French nobles into trying Asian ginseng as a cure for exhaustion and impotence. Now ginseng's New World connection became the buzz of the royal court. Merchants were thrilled that the colonies offered a trade complement to furs. When Lafitau's botanical samples arrived in Paris, the Royal Academy erupted with speculation about the exact relationship between Asian and American ginseng, and with arguments over Lafitau's hypothesis that the similarity of the plant's Iroquois and Chinese names signaled a historical link between Asia and America. The scientific debate jumped the English Channel and consumed London as well, but a commercial scramble quickly overwhelmed the academic questions. By 1724 English colonials in New York were digging ginseng and sending samples to London for analysis. Ginseng added fuel to the feverish competition between the French and the British for the fur trade. In America, the fortunes of ginseng would now be linked, through generations of trappers and traders, with the hides of fur-bearing creatures.

LAFITAU'S DISCOVERY HAD AN immediate effect in Canada. All through the summer of 1716, the Iroquois of Montreal made good money selling ginseng to French merchants for shipments to China. A Swede visiting Canada wrote that Indians were scouring the forest for the root, and the ones in his neighborhood were so busy digging ginseng that French farmers couldn't find anyone to hire for regular farm work. Soon colonists were learning how to find it, too, and the plant that Lafitau had said was abundant near Montreal became almost extinct there. The Iroquois had to venture far into the English colonies to dig enough for the French merchants of La Rochelle.

"There was a ginseng frenzy in New France," according to Andreas Motsch, a Lafitau scholar at the University of Montreal. By 1752, Canada's ginseng exports amounted to half a million francs a year. And Canada's forests would soon be stripped clean. Other New World discoveries have brought more destructive transformations. The discovery of rubber, for instance, triggered a boom that ripped through South America in the 1800s, claiming the lives of nearly half of Brazil's indigenous population and entirely extinguishing dozens of ethnic groups. Rubber barons turned villages into private fiefdoms and sent them deep into malaria-ridden forests to tap more and more rubber trees. Compared to that, the rush for ginseng was benign.

Meanwhile Lafitau remained stuck in France, swamped in administrative chores. In 1724 he published a massive work on North American Indians. He compared their customs with the ancient Greeks and Romans, citing over two hundred sources, from Boetius, Casaubon, and Herodotus to Homer, Ovid, Plato, Plutarch, Socrates, Tacitus, Virgil, and Xenophon. His writing style was awkward and off-putting, and a contemporary reviewer found the work too long, confusing, and hard to read. The book sank almost without a trace.

So at age forty-six Lafitau returned to Canada to lead the Montreal mission, apparently glad to go. He stayed there for several years and then retired to his hometown of Bordeaux, where he died. In his lifetime he was dismissed by other intellectuals. Voltaire mocked Lafitau's theory of a link between Native Americans and the ancient Greeks:

> [Lafitau] would derive the Americans from the ancient Greeks and these are his reasons: The Greeks have myths; some Americans have them too. The first Greeks went hunting; the Americans go too. The first Greeks had oracles; the Americans have sorcerers. In the festivals of Greece there was dancing; there is dancing in America. It must be avowed that these reasons are convincing.

Lafitau's system for comparing cultures was ignored for most of a century, but by the early 1800s German scholars had discovered his work. He was called the "first of the modern ethnographers and a precursor of scientific ethnology," and a founder of anthropology. The idea of an ancient link between Asia and the Americas is no longer ridiculed. It's accepted. But more than that, every fall his living legacy is found in the thousands of diggers who fan out into forests across eastern North America, searching for a plant.

FIVE

Pursued by Trappers

*As a Help to bear Fatigue, I us'd to chew a
Root of Ginseng as I Walk't along. That kept up my Spirits,
and made me trip away as nimbly in my Jack-Boots as
younger men cou'd in their Shoes.*

—WILLIAM BYRD, Virginia colonial propagandist (1674–1744)

A<small>S</small> S<small>EPTEMBER ADVANCED</small> I followed the fall colors to West Virginia. The Mountain State is one of the largest exporters of wild American ginseng and a place where the country's digging history still lives in the present. Approaching Charleston, I looked out the airplane window at the misty valleys and mountaintops, many of them bald with angular clearings that resembled fairways—strip mines replanted with grass.

In West Virginia I arranged to meet up with Dave Cooke, an agricultural agent, in the parking lot of a Magic Mart off Route 119. A year before, Cooke had introduced me to George Albright and several other ginsengers. Ginsengers could be hard for an outsider to find, owing to the need for secrecy. "The way it's been in the past, if somebody finds out you got ginseng on your land, it disappears," one West Virginia digger explained. "It's like having money buried on your property."

During that first visit George had taken me and Cooke to hunt ginseng in his woods. George had pointed out the signs of good ginseng habitat and the indicator plants he looked for: sarsaparilla, cohosh, certain kinds of ferns, bloodroot, mayapple. He showed me other things too, like how a handful of minerals could attract deer (he called the mixture "deer cocaine"), and beneath the canopy of maples and poplars, he demonstrated his digging technique. He started nearly a foot away from the stem, to avoid cutting the root, "because it might be going up the hill, you don't know which way it's laying." George had scraped the soil surface with a pick and a degree of respect worthy of a Manchu digger. "You don't know which way it's laying," he had repeated, almost to himself.

As I sat in front of the Magic Mart waiting for Cooke, I recalled George's concentration and wondered if there was something almost primordial in ginseng's allure. In *The Botany of Desire,* Michael Pollan suggests that, in evolutionary terms, a plant may use its desirability to dispersal agents—including humans—to increase its population as widely as possible through the world. Apples, for example, were once native only to western Asia, but their taste and appeal to people through the ages had spread them to every continent. Pollan was talking about plants that humans have cultivated for thousands of years—apples, tulips, potatoes, and marijuana. But ginseng had resisted cultivation for a long time—its requirements for shade and soil are too particular for most farms. Yet its chemistry or its shape made it a particular prize for people where it grew: indigenous groups in both Asia and North America had helped to replenish it (alongside other plants they valued) in the forest.

Beyond that, could a wild plant's survival power snowball as it gained economic and cultural importance? After several thousand years of use in China, ginseng's reputation as a medicinal tonic gave it a value so high that it financed Nurhaci's gambit to take over an empire in the seventeenth century. Nurhaci took what was merely a valuable medicinal plant and turned it into an item of cultural identity for the Manchus. Their monopoly on its trade boosted ginseng's status even more throughout Qing-era China and increased the likelihood that foreigners like Father Jartoux would notice the plant during his travels for the atlas and write home about it. Ginseng's significance in Appalachian culture today is thus a direct result of its cultural importance in Asia. Although that has caused wild American ginseng to be dug nearly to extinction in some states, it has generally helped increase the plant's global population, mainly through commercial farming. Ginseng has been cultivated, or at least attempted, on every continent except Antarctica.

From a plant's perspective, Pollan argues, it doesn't really matter whether it survives as wild or cultivated, as long as the species survives in the long haul. A widespread population helps, and so does a genetic base broad enough to handle the challenges of new viruses and disease. That's where infusions of genetic variation from the wild are important; even common crops need the varied genetic resources of their wild relatives for adapting to new climates and new diseases. If ginseng's wild populations disappeared, its ability to come up with new genetic combinations would be diminished and with that, its ability to adapt. Yet with people like Bob Beyfuss gathering wild samples of American ginseng seed from throughout its native range and saving that variety, and with farmers planting the root far and wide, ginseng may be *gaining* resources for long-term survival, despite its endangered label. It's hard to tell.

In a more subtle way, it might also be true that ginseng gains resilience by attracting different elements of human society—not just people involved in medicine, but also in culture and commerce. Plants that have adapted to several ecosystems have more flexibility to survive climatic changes; in the same way, maybe a plant that has niches in several societies is more adaptable. Ginseng harvests in China became more important when Nurhaci, a person with direct, rural knowledge of ginseng, moved to the center of Chinese society. Yet without someone in America familiar with the Jesuit experience in China, it's unlikely that American ginseng would ever have become an international item. Making the leap from knowing about a valuable Chinese plant to finding it in America's forests probably required a scholar like Lafitau (and a copy of the Jesuit newsletter). It also required his knowledge of Native American culture. Furthermore, Lafitau's information on ginseng in North America could have remained an obscure bit of academic trivia tucked in the Duke of Orleans' library if merchants hadn't taken up the baton. A plant's cultural habitats—the communities where it lives in stories of large 'sang patches, cash payoffs, and botanical novelties—could become a field of study itself.

For the wild heart of the ginseng culture, West Virginia is a good place to look. Some of the liveliest stories about ginseng originated there, including several involving Daniel Boone, the

prototypical American woodsman. Boone embodied the over-
lapping histories of ginsenging and fur trapping and trading.
One of the most popular stories, featured everywhere from
Fur-Fish-Game magazine to the Discovery Channel, tells of
Boone and his barge of ginseng. One fall, the story goes, he
worked hard digging ginseng and buying more and more until he had a bargeload full of roots ready to take to market. But
as he was crossing the Ohio River from Kentucky to Point
Pleasant, the barge swamped. Instead of despairing, Boone
commissioned men to go out and dig more ginseng. The episode said something both about ginseng's enduring value and
Boone's perseverance.

BEFORE LONG DAVE COOKE appeared at the Magic
Mart. Cooke is tall and rangy, and his collar-length hair and
white-streaked goatee give him a Buffalo Bill–style panache. He
was born in nearby Lincoln County to a mining family. "Where
we came from there were two sources of income," Cooke told
me, "you had ginseng and moonshine." When Dave was four,
his father was injured in the mines and the family moved to
Huntington. Dave's older brother recalled digging 'sang with
their father, but Dave was raised in town. He grew up, moved
away, married, worked as a furniture maker in Florida, divorced,
and then came back to Appalachia. He didn't learn about the
woods or ginseng until he was forty.

His job as an extension agent in the state's agricultural system
meant that he covered four counties, giving people advice on
everything from livestock to nutrition. Dave was also the official
state resource on ginseng. In that capacity he gave workshops

around West Virginia and answered questions from would-be ginseng growers. Cooke described himself as "just an old redneck boy, a coal miner's son," but that's partly a matter of positioning for his audience. At other times he called himself a "reverted hippie."

In the year since our first meeting, Cooke had remarried and moved out of his home on Big Ugly Creek to his wife's house by the four-lane. When I met him at the Magic Mart he looked tired and sounded congested. "This cold is kicking my ass," he said. He had also just learned that his 4-H coordinator was leaving, which meant that Cooke would have to stack another job onto his full workload for at least six months. And he had left the chemistry kit for testing fishponds at his office, so he had to pick that up. We'd be late for our meeting with George.

Like Bob Beyfuss, Dave Cooke took ginseng occasionally when he felt a little ragged. Despite the terrible taste, which he described as resembling an extremely bitter carrot, he mixed thin slices of the root in a glass of water and drank it down. Overall, he was more interested in ginseng's promise of income for rural families than in its medicinal value. Cooke preached the root's potential as a moneymaker for West Virginian families. He told me that while folks all through Lincoln County relied on ginseng for their kids' school clothes and Christmas presents, he wanted to make ginseng more than just an occasional digging expedition.

"We're constantly fighting what I call the corn-and-bean mentality," he told me once. That mentality says, If you can't get a crop out of the ground in ninety to a hundred and twenty days, and sell it, why do it? The bias toward short-rotation crops

gave short shrift to longer-term enterprises like ginseng growing. Cooke once compared the state's investment in beef cattle,
which are not suited to its mountain slopes and forest land, with
its investment in ginseng, which is native to both. Support for
the cattle industry was many times greater than support for ginseng. The state dedicated fifty to sixty employees full-time to
beef cattle, along with facilities like auction barns, weighing in-
stallations, and county fairgrounds that supported beef-cattle
farms. To ginseng, it allocated just one part-time expert: Dave
Cooke. Yet the state's exports of beef cattle were just four times
its ginseng exports. The disparity, Cooke felt, was glaring.

Cooke, like Beyfuss, fulminated against an unthinking agriculture that he considered poorly adapted to mountains. But
living against a more dire background, Cooke gave vivid and
apocalyptic sermons that turned on a cycle of logging and coal.
Arguably the most famous image of Boone County, where
Cooke lived, was *The Dancing Outlaw,* a 1991 cult documentary
about a white-trash Elvis impersonator/clogger and his family.
The local unemployment rate was roughly twice the national
average, and a quarter of the county's families lived below the
poverty level.

"I'm seeing this right now, driving out of my holler on Big
Ugly," he told me once. "It used to be everybody who lived on
that holler, somebody in that family worked in the coal mines.
That's not the case now. But I'm seeing hills over there that
look like they've been hit by tornadoes, because the loggers are
coming back. You see this every couple of generations all
through this part of Appalachia. And we're seeing it very pow-
erfully now."

On the other hand, Boone County still had a lot of ginseng-friendly forest. The technical classification of "mixed mesophytic" meant that it was a rare relic of the old forest that once covered Laurasia: hickories and oaks in the valleys, and maples, hemlock, and mountain laurel higher up the slopes. The tradition of ginsenging for extra cash was still alive here. Boone County was the third-highest ginseng-producing county in the state. In the 1990s a field researcher from the Library of Congress found plenty of residents who identified themselves as 'sangers. "I make my living in construction," one man said, "but really, I consider myself a ginsenger." His philosophy combined self-reliance and a knowledge of the woods: "Don't lay around on your deadbeat ass and get a check from the government. There's ginseng, there's bloodroot, there's yellowroot."

You might think that people in Boone County would fill Cooke's seminars on how to make more money with ginseng. When he gave workshops in Ohio, Virginia, and elsewhere, they drew a wide range of old and young, men and women, people who knew the woods well and not at all. He got retirees, New Age holistic-health practitioners, old hippies, and many "practical, hardheaded people." He got calls from men who hauled water by hand uphill to grow ginseng in their woods, and from a husband-and-wife team who planted whole hillsides with root. (West Virginia may have proportionally more women ginsengers than New York. Local journals include stories of mother-daughter 'sang hunts.) People asked him about regulations governing ginseng. When the U.S. Fish and Wildlife Service announced that wild ginseng roots under five years old would be seized at the export docks, Cooke said, "I had people calling me on the phone in tears. I had people calling me cursing." (That law, intended to spare young ginseng plants from harvest pressures, proved difficult to enforce.)

Yet folks locally didn't come out for his workshops. Maybe they thought they already knew about ginseng, or maybe they just didn't go for workshops. A local ginseng dealer, one of the biggest in the county who also ran a fee-fishing operation off Six-Mile Road, came to one workshop just to disrupt it.

"He just thinks I'm full of shit," Cooke said. "He wants to keep things quiet. He doesn't want anybody to know any more about it than they do." The buyer walked up to a table where Cooke had laid out a variety of unlabeled ginseng roots to illustrate different ages and growing conditions. With a flourish, he confidently identified each one.

"He got every one of them wrong," Cooke said. "With absolute certainty. I just let him get his spleen out, and he left. And then we got on with the workshop. Guys like that you can't talk with."

Cooke also knew you couldn't lead a ginseng workshop the way you teach a seminar on the university's main campus. Farmers would laugh at you and walk out. Printed handouts are almost useless, since many who show up are functionally illiterate. So Cooke made what he calls his "corny little ginseng video," a twenty-minute introduction to wild-simulated 'sang that shows Cooke in the woods sowing, planting, and harvesting. He has given out hundreds of copies of that tape and even had it dubbed in Mandarin for viewers in China. ("They thought that was too funny for words," he said.) He wants to make an updated, longer version with an accompanying CD.

Cooke's efforts to inform growers about the market often met with resistance from ginseng buyers and traders. Dealers have always had a strong interest in keeping ginseng's price secret. Through the years their profit margin remained healthy if the people who gathered the root in Appalachia, where the plant was abundant, didn't know what consumers paid for it in China, where it was rare. Generations of diggers had no leverage for getting a better price for their ginseng, because they had no clue about its market value in Hong Kong. They were selling their root blind.

Given these problems where ginseng grows naturally, Cooke was amused at how much effort people outside the plant's native range put into growing it. Farmers in the Pacific Northwest have planted tons of root, and so have growers in Arizona. There was even a man growing it in Australia. "There's something wrong with that guy in the head," Cooke said, noting Australia's forbiddingly dry climate. "But now he's got a big, big market."

From the Magic Mart we drove beside a winding stream to where the road ended in gravel. Yellow posted signs were wrapped around tree trunks, and a big plywood sign announced in red letters:

POSTED

STAY OUT!

GEORGE ALBRIGHT

We passed the gate and drove to the far end of a clearing, to a house near the edge of the woods. George Albright kept a tidy one-story ranch house. Inside he had the living-room TV tuned to MSNBC.

Albright combined the ginsenger tradition with the information savvy of a new breed. He was thin, his hair and beard were a pale blond, and his eyes were an unsettling blue. Dave Cooke described him as "lean and kind of greyhound-looking." For decades, George operated the hydraulics equipment that served the mining industry in five states ("They got big shovels that you could park off two or three automobiles in," he told me). After retiring, he returned to these woods, near where he had learned to dig 'sang over fifty years ago, and brought back an eye for market trends. Besides ginseng, George tinkered with markets from wildflowers to butterflies. This morning he asked Cooke about the bullfrog market, which he had read about. Bullfrogs require investments in fencing, lights, and feed, Cooke explained, but if George was interested he knew where to buy tadpoles. These two were checking angles on a rural economy I hadn't dreamt of.

They were mulling over an awareness of the land that was increasingly scarce, one sustained through generations by people making a living from sweat, soil, and the vagaries of nature. Their talk was a reminder that such knowledge has often been saved at higher elevations. Around the world, mountains shelter vanishing cultural traditions as well as rare plants and wildlife. Upland areas have a greater variety of species than lowlands because they have more varied habitats—more niches of differing moisture, temperature, and sunlight. Plant life and the colors of autumn vary from one valley to the next, and from the east face of a mountain to its west side. These hills likewise have given refuge to people who don't find a niche in mainstream society. Another West Virginian I met described his theory of how topography influenced the state's social history. The eastern half of the state, hatched by straight ridges and valleys, was easily settled in the 1700s by marginalized groups like the Mennonites. The more remote and serpentine ridges of the western half attracted idiosyncratic latecomers, including snake-handling sects and loners. The obstacles of terrain shaped the contours of life for people as well as plants.

"Bullfrog legs are expensive," George said, still weighing the options.

Back in the 1980s, before Dave Cooke started coming around, Albright started seeding ginseng in his own woods. But he rarely uses the awkward term "simulated-wild."

"I had ginsenged all my life," George said, "and I just got it in my head I wanted to do it." He bought seed from Paul Hsu in Wisconsin and dropped it along the bottomlands beside a creek, beneath poplar and sycamore, because he had dug root under that mixture of trees before.

So far this season he hadn't dug much ginseng but he'd scouted a few spots. From year to year he tracked ginseng on his own land and on various parcels around town—near a school, beside a path he takes to the grocery store. "There's one patch right across the creek up here," he said. "The year I had surgery, I found a little patch up there. But every year I go back to check and that ginseng's not there. And I marked it! I haven't been by there this year but I'm going to wait. It's stirring me. I'm going to wait one more year . . ."

It was George who told Cooke about ginseng's ability to stay dormant for years on end with no sign of it aboveground. He studied it this way and memorized its points in the landscape. He talked of one spot in the woods that had its own season. "Right here on the hill, the road goes to a fork. In May the phlox are blue, they grow about this tall, about twelve inches, geraniums are pink," he said emphatically. "The mountain is just a blanket of flowers just as far as you can see. It's one of the most beautiful sights you ever seen in your life. May. Absolutely beautiful."

Growing up in the woods, George hunted and trapped, and when somebody killed a groundhog he was sent to fetch spice-bush twigs, which his mother would cook with the groundhog "to take the wild taste out of it." When he was about twelve, he learned to dig ginseng from his father and friends. They also dug goldenseal, which people there called yellowroot. When George had a cold his mother would make a yellowroot tea for him to gargle. He figured the horrible taste just distracted him from the sore throat. "It's bitter, ain't it, Dave? Lord have mercy."

When George said he lived twenty-eight years at the edge of the city, he was referring to Logan, population under fifty thousand. He was one of the most informed and curious people I've ever met, tracking changes in the laws that affected him and holding opinions on them, including the new Fish and Wildlife rule that banned harvests of roots under five years old. (He regarded the law as well-intentioned but probably not effective at reducing the harvest of young ginseng. In 2005, the agency raised the minimum age to ten years.) When he saw a plant he didn't know, he went straight to his plant book. "I'm just that type," he said. "I love the outdoors." Every time I visited him, he had just found a new plant that he was trying to identify.

George was wary of loggers, saying they routinely took advantage of people and ignored the rules a landowner gave them about the limits of their harvest. They often cut trees beyond the boundaries set out, or they clear-cut areas where they were told to cut selectively. If loggers found a ginseng patch, George said, the boss would give them a ten-minute break to dig it out.

One particular patch still tugged at his heart. He found it on his neighbor's land after loggers had cleared it. "They went up there, cut timber, took it over and just tore it open," he said. "I dug about a pound in about four hours, which is very good. It seemed like every treetop where they'd been through and the tree was dying, I'd find big ginseng. I found a log that was topped, it fell on this ginseng. There was three-, four-prong . . . The log was laying like this and the ginseng was growing out from under the logs. I was under this log a-digging, and I turn around and looked. And here was a big four-prong about that tall." He put his hand out about three feet high. "Berries. If I hadn't just looked up and saw those berries, I never would have found that four-prong.

"But you run into a lot of things," he went on. "You find some place where you don't think there should be any ginseng, there's all kinds of it there."

Our conversation moved on to other things, but later George circled back to that logging site. "When I saw that big one, it made cold tears go over me when I got up and looked at it. I'd give anything if I'd had my camera. I'd give *anything* if I'd had my camera that day."

• • •

GEORGE ALSO HAD EXPERTISE with ginseng dealers. There are two types of dealer, he said: One type runs a local business—a recycling shop, for example, or a bait-and-tackle shop—and buys people's ginseng on the side, usually small amounts. He usually doesn't pay the highest price, but he's convenient because he's nearby. The second type comes around year after year during the fall, a circuit rider: he pays more but you don't know when you'll see him next. When George was a boy, a man would pass through this part of the state with a thick roll of hundred-dollar bills in his bib overalls. People in towns up and down the Big Coal River recall Giles the 'sang man coming around on foot. People in Peytona say he was a big man with a dark beard. He might start walking in Whitesville and cover over twenty miles in a day, buying ginseng along the way. He could spend the night anywhere darkness caught him. He might look like a bum but he would show local boys one of his C-notes and call it his pocket change. His nearest counterpart these days is a guy in Huntington, an hour and a half away, who comes through during the season.

George didn't sell his roots to just anybody. He checked the newspaper, where buyers advertise, and shopped around for the best price. In magazines like *Fur-Fish-Game* you find classifieds like this:

> Wanted: Dealers and diggers of Ginseng, Goldenseal, Kansas Snake Root, Sassafras, Root Bark and others. We are direct buyers of ginseng for the Chinese. Ship Parcel Post or UPS. Send SASE, including phone number to: Hammond's Fur, Hide & Root Co., 3050 E. Ramp Creek Dr., Bloomington, IN 47401

As we talked, George's year-old gray cat prowled the porch. "Ground moles, ground squirrels, she brings everything in," he said. "She's a hunter, all right."

When we started talking about poaching, George's mood darkened noticeably. He complained that people don't pay attention to his POSTED signs. He had to run off six or eight people already this year. This led the conversation crabwise to a story about Chicken Charley, a neighbor with family problems and who drank. When three of George's patches of ginseng walked away, George intended to find out who was responsible. He suspected Charley. "The reason they call him Chicken Charley was, he'd go up here and steal this boy's chickens off the roost. Yeah, he would. I was standing up there ginsenging, and I was taking a break. And here he comes walking around the hill, looking like . . . I guess looking for pot or something." (Dave Cooke interjected that marijuana was one of the biggest sources of cash income in the county.) "I said, 'What do you say, Charley?' He jumped. He said, 'What are you doing?' I said, 'What are *you* doing?'

"He said, 'I was just looking around.'

"I said, 'Go back and look th' other way.' I said, 'It's posted, you don't need to be looking up here.' I knew what he was doing. He had found my ginseng. I had the first three patches up, I had planted two years in a row, and he got every bit of it."

You could still hear the outrage in George's voice. Yes, there are laws on the books against ginseng theft, but state agencies rarely prosecute. "The enforcement sucks," Dave Cooke said. By this point we had walked out past George's blackberry bushes to his fishpond, where he hoped to raise bullfrogs.

George waded into the pond and hauled a cylindrical wooden trap from the water. He dumped its contents on the grass—a bunch of pesky crawfish—and, still furious, began to stomp them with his boots until they crunched underfoot.

"Look at all that food he's squashing!" Dave said in mock horror.

"Food!" George said sarcastically.

LIKE DANIEL BOONE, George combined the skills of a ginsenger with those of a trapper, and Albright often sold his ginseng through contacts in the fur trade. Most dealers traded in both; they bought ginseng in the fall and furs in the winter. They sold furs through one channel and exported ginseng through another. The fur trade had created a closed network for ginseng, controlled largely by New York furriers. (That may be why trappers cared more about ginseng than foresters, and why now it's tracked by the Fish and Wildlife Service, not the Forest Service. Foresters rarely bothered with ginseng, apart from the logging crews that would dig out your patches when you hired them to cut your timber.) Through the twentieth century, fur prices fell and ginseng prices rose. When the fur industry finally tanked in the early 1980s—brought down in good measure by changing ideas about animal rights—the seasonal symbiosis disappeared. But those ties remain visible in the West Virginia Trappers Association.

About a dozen years ago George went to a fur-and-root auction organized by the trappers association. The auction is a biannual event at which brokers come to bid and ginsengers and trappers come to sell. The fall auction is just for plant material (roots, bark, and leaves); the one in winter sells both plants and fur. For that one, held at a community center or a racetrack (George couldn't recall for sure), he went with his younger son, then a teenager, who one summer had made six hundred dollars digging 'sang and trapping muskrats. They planned to make the two-hour drive to the auction, sell their ginseng, and get home on the early side.

"You walk in and there's a smell like nothing you ever smelled," said Cooke, who had been to several auctions himself. "Raw, dried fur. Literally thousands and thousands of hides. Everything from muskrat and bobcat to wolf . . . Bear. Everything you could think of." Some of the people look like Grizzly Adams, some reportedly come out of the hills only for the auction or to buy salt and coffee.

"They've got their own clothes they've made out of their furs," George said. "They'd sell everything. They make knives out of deerhorn. They're mountain men. Play guitar, sit there and play a banjo." The spectacle held George spellbound. In the auction they got top price for their ginseng. He and his son ended up staying the whole day, just watching people.

As we talked, the bad taste from the poaching discussion was fading. "They had a pile of ginseng about that deep! These guys bring their instruments. They sit, pick, and sing. I really enjoyed it," George said.

"It would be good to go back," he added. Then he turned to Cooke. "When did you say it's going to be?"

GINSENG'S DEEP CONNECTIONS with fur traders spawned legends that gave it animal characteristics and intelligence.

Taxonomies of plant and animal life are clear and reasonable, but they are, after all, artificial frameworks for understanding a complicated world. When André Michaux, a French botanist of the 1700s and a strong ginseng advocate, wanted information about plants on the frontier, he sought out fur trappers. If you spend a lot of time looking for wildlife, he reasoned, you'll also know the plants. In some ways, ginseng has more in common with deer than it does with walnut trees. It certainly has a more intimate relationship with deer, which browse on ginseng's leaves and berries. The ginseng seeds wind their way through the deer's digestive organs and get dispersed to new sites in the animal's droppings. The bonds of survival cross over the borders of taxonomy.

Daniel Boone and his friend Paddy Huddleston were the first colonists to trap beavers in the Kanawha River valley above Charleston, and hunted ginseng there too. For years, they sold beaver pelts to dealers in Philadelphia. Huddleston ran an inn upriver in the town of Alloy. By then Boone was already famous thanks to a biography published in 1784, when he was fifty years old, that portrayed him as a swashbuckling frontiersman. Boone himself was more modest. When asked if he had ever been lost in the woods, he answered, "I was never lost, but I was bewildered once for three days." Just as that biography made him famous, Boone's fortunes suffered a downward spiral. His businesses and attempts at land speculation failed. When he came to the Kanawha valley in the late 1780s, he was looking for the next big thing.

Judging by reports in newspapers then, the next big thing might be ginseng. Boone had dug ginseng for years before the

Revolution, but when the war started he and other ginsengers lost access to the China-bound British ships. Soon after the war ended, the *Empress of China* became the first American ship to venture to the Far East, and returned to New York harbor with tales of a strong market for American ginseng. So the winter of 1787 found Daniel Boone digging hard and buying up other people's root, too. His son Nathan was just six years old, but big enough to camp out and help with the digging. "By the next spring we had some twelve or fifteen tons," Nathan recalled later. He estimated his father trapped four or five hundred beaver pelts every winter and sold them for about $2.50 each. That meant over a thousand dollars for a winter's work of rubbing sticks with castor bait and sticking them into the banks of Limestone Creek. Boone could dig ginseng in the fall while scouting the best terrain for winter trapping sites.

He planned to take his ginseng cargo up the Ohio River in the spring to Wheeling, where he could pack it on horses along the Wilderness Road to Hagerstown, Maryland. From there they could take a main route to Philadelphia, the port for ships going to the Far East. Walking through Philadelphia then, you could see the city's new wealth from the China trade in the homes of merchants on Walnut Street, and in shops that sold porcelain, crystallized ginger candy, and Chinese cinnamon. More and more men were wearing work trousers made from nankeen, a sturdy yellowish cotton fabric (the name came from Nanking, the cloth's home port). By the late 1780s even George Washington, who always had a weather eye out for enterprise, tracked ginseng as it moved from the hills to the docks. "I met numbers of Persons & Pack horses going in with Ginsang," he wrote in his journal of a trip through the Appalachians one autumn, "& for salt & other articles at the Markets below . . ."

Following Boone's trail, I drove downriver from Charleston, beside the Kanawha's flat water as it cut through a wide valley of cornfields. Where it flowed into the Ohio River, I crossed a metal bridge into the town of Point Pleasant and found the spot, just beyond on Route 2, where Boone's trading post had stood, now commemorated by a roadside marker. In the park nearby two FedEx drivers took a break from the last of the summer heat. There was still a ginseng dealer in town, but these days she lived in a one-story suburban home with a massive rhododendron bush.

The front desk clerk at the old Lowe Hotel on the waterfront told me about Point Pleasant's heyday as a transport hub for traffic on the Ohio River, and that the hotel had been a popular riverboat stop in the early 1800s. His name was Rush and he was in a conversational mood. He explained how George Washington had named the town and envisioned it as a future nation's capital, facing a westward trade. Rush talked about Daniel Boone's trading post, and confirmed that ginseng still grew wild locally but higher up, in the dark hollers. He had dug 'sang as a kid. He told me about Mark Twain's grandfather and namesake, Samuel Clemens, who lived in Point Pleasant as a tax collector and was killed at a house-raising here under questionable circumstances. (There was no evident link to ginseng in the death, but Twain's father dealt in 'sang when he ran a general store in Tennessee.) Rush voiced strong opinions about why Simon Kenton, not Boone, should be called the father of Kentucky, and he offered advice on how to float a raft down rapids:

portage the cargo, loosen the raft's lashing to let the logs absorb the shocks, let it go and recapture it downstream, retighten the lashings, and reload the cargo. He enumerated the advantages of river travel over land travel (cleaner and faster; on deeply rutted roads, horses slogged nearly up to their bellies in mud), assessed the state's best farm country (here), and affirmed the beauty of the Shenandoah.

I walked outside and stood in a park at the point where the two rivers meet, looking out across the Ohio. Two tugboats passed, and to my left the late sun struck the bridge over the Kanawha, against inky storm clouds beyond. To my right the Ohio flowed to where the land seemed to spread wider and flatter.

This was where Boone's keelboat full of ginseng ran into trouble. He and his family were crossing the Ohio River just a few hundred yards upstream from Point Pleasant when the powerful current pushed them onto driftwood. The barge tipped and filled with water. No lives were lost, but the tons of ginseng were ruined. The family sent a runner into town for help, and when a friend of Boone's arrived, they spread the roots out on the shore to dry. But the damage was done. "Father didn't get half the regular price," Nathan recalled. Worse, the delay meant that the ginseng reached Philadelphia after the price had tumbled. "Father lost money by the operation."

So the story of Daniel Boone's ginseng barge, routinely cited as a case of ginseng's enduring marketability, showed instead that ginseng has always been a risky business. Even when ginseng was a good bet, it could be more of a gamble than Dave Cooke or Bob Beyfuss might want to admit.

• • •

To MAKE GINSENG a more reliable enterprise for growers, Dave Cooke needed better information on the market in China. In 1996, that meant going with two other extension agents to China, supported by the U.S. Department of Agriculture. Amazingly, no agency had ever before sought direct knowledge of the ginseng market, even though it had once been a leading U.S. export. Since the early twentieth century, the plant had remained in a backwater of officialdom. Mechanized agriculture for field crops and dairy cattle grew more profitable than furs or medicinal plants. Information on the ginseng market grew scarce. Even lifelong diggers knew almost nothing about what their end-customers really wanted—what size roots, or color, or texture. Few ginsengers had ever met a person who bought ginseng for their own use. So ginsengers would stop by Cooke's house and excitedly show him their harvest: a huge root with its neck broken off. "This is a decades-old root—valuable!—and they've cut its market value at the end-user by fifty percent," he told me with exasperation.

Cooke and two other county agents made the seventeen-hour, world-spanning flight from Charleston's Chuck Yeager Airport to Beijing. From there they were whisked to northeastern China, the home of Asian ginseng, formerly known as Manchuria. Their first stop was Shenyang, Nurhaci's old capital. In the countryside, jet lag amplified the disorienting sensation of undoing continental drift.

"There's that band through northeast China that has the same mesophytic temperate, mixed-hardwood forest that we do," Cooke explained to me. "So it was really cool to walk through what woods we could see. If you'd squint just a little bit, it was like being here. The oak trees, the hickory trees, the poplars, the walnuts. They were *slightly* different—it was a mandarin walnut as opposed to a black walnut—but it was so close."

Further north, near Jilin City, they looked out on five hundred acres of cultivated American ginseng growing under artificial shade, monitored by a squad of more than two dozen scientists who handled plant breeding, physiology, and processing. Their hosts asked the three Americans, How many Ph.D.s are working on ginseng back where you come from?

Cooke recalls that moment clearly. "We just looked at each other." There wasn't a Ph.D. among them. "They persisted in calling us 'doctor.' I'm about as far from a doctor as you could hope." It was a vivid reminder of the differences between the two countries. Here ginseng was an unrefined product; in China it *was* agribusiness.

From George Albright's place, Cooke pointed me toward my next rendezvous, in another parking lot, this time east of Charleston. Fred Hays, I knew, would be an excellent guide to where old ginsenging skills came up against new realities. Hays ran a "holistic farm." He was a younger entrepreneur, and spoke more plainly than Cooke or George Albright about a coming conflict between urban and rural attitudes. Fred had offered to take me 'sang hunting on his land, and met me just off the interstate. I followed him to his place. Where Dave Cooke could riff easily on many topics, Fred chose his words carefully. With short reddish hair and a few days' growth on his jaw, he had the air of a big teddy bear.

In a way, Fred embodied several types of people who went into simulated-wild ginseng, which he described as a "growing movement." It attracted mountain men as well as back-to-the-landers from the suburbs. He himself grew up here in the Kanawha valley but went to college, a fact that by itself put him between cultures. "There's people up and down this road," he told me, "that if you went to college, they don't trust you." He was a farmer but also a professional artist whose wife was trained in psychotherapy. Fred met Bob Beyfuss at a ginseng conference that Beyfuss hosted several years before and had seen Beyfuss go through a tough divorce. They kept in touch by e-mail, and Fred let the older man dig roots on his land. "Bob's a pretty down-to-earth guy," Fred said. "He fit right in here."

Fred's holistic farm covers a hundred and fifty acres and includes a fishpond and a grassy slope where goats were grazing, as well as many acres under forest. As he adjusted the goats' tethers so they wouldn't tangle, he explained his new effort at timber-stand improvement, which involved mapping every single tree in his forest, pruning out unwanted newcomers and freeing desirable native tree species to grow. Hays combined that native-tree approach with growing simulated-wild ginseng under the forest canopy.

On a porch overlooking the fishpond, he told stories of hunting 'sang that tended to be more deadly than George Albright's. For instance: "One of ginseng's favorite places is very rocky areas. That's also where rattlesnakes are. And if ginseng's out, so are rattlesnakes. I was at a place the summer before last, and I spotted some big ginseng but there were two boulders the size of this house, with a gap about five feet wide between them.

And you had to go through there or you weren't getting out, because it was straight up and down everywhere else. I started through there and saw a rattlesnake. He was almost five feet long, reared up waist-high in front of me, started rattling. It was either me or him. I've got his hide over at the house.

"The worst are the copperheads. They're silent," he said. "When you dig wild ginseng, you've got to have along protection."

Fred learned ginseng from his father, who learned from *his* father's brother, an old-style mountain man who knew everything about ginseng, hunting, tracking, how to trap muskrats and mink, the whole ball of wax. Fred's great-uncle was the kind that stayed in the hills all winter and lived off the land without cash crops like tobacco or corn. "There was a season for everything. They dug ginseng, they trapped fur, and they made ends meet that way."

Fred knew animals as friend and foe, with the intimacy of a cranky neighbor. He had watched their behavior all his life and he had problems with some of their antics, for example when mink killed the fish in his pond for sport. "They don't take one fish out and eat it," he complained, "they spend all night taking *every* fish out of the cage and piling them on the dock, just letting them flop and die. You'll go up and there will be a hundred fish laying there." He imitated a mink catching a fish and tossing it aside, already bored. "Wow! Look at all these fish!"

He paid his way through college as a ginseng digger and a trapper. Back then a red fox hide sold for $120, he could dig a pound of ginseng in a day, and he could sell both nearby. He found it ironic that fur became such a dirty word, as if we're all better off wearing polymers made from crude oil.

He saw a culture clash coming. Back-to-the-landers were bringing new ideas of ecological farming and landscapes to the country. They give new names to old plants: rattleweed becomes black cohosh (and, incidentally, a chichi garden plant). Yellowroot becomes goldenseal. The urbanites bring weapons against which mountain people are especially vulnerable, like bureaucracy. Back-to-the-landers, Fred said, "are more social than rural people. That's not the correct word. They end up on local council boards and all that kind of stuff, and they start making policies for you." *Policies* sounded particularly disgusting. "They seem to come from the city with the idea that they're coming here to save the environment from the heathen who are already here. And then they eventually become one of them and realize they weren't such heathen after all."

He thought the next ten or twenty years would be critical. "I can see it as headline news at some point. We're on a collision course. It's going to be: 'Urban America Goes to Rural America.' And how are they going to live together? It's almost like different races."

Ginseng offered him a rare bright spot; in it, he saw economic promise for rural people and an incentive for wiser use of forests. "Ginseng is a survivor," he said. "If there's one plant out there that would be hard to make extinct, it would be ginseng." He viewed the plant's dormancy behavior as a way to get through bad times. After neighbors up the road had their timber cut several years before, Fred walked through and found an ancient ginseng plant waist-high. It was seventy years old. "Seventy notches on the roots. It had probably been hiding for forty years, come up once every ten years or so. There's a lot more ginseng there than people are ever going to find."

FRED'S STORIES OF GINSENG traders were nearly as harrowing as his rattlesnake tales. The local 'sang and fur dealer when Hays was a boy was Old Man Naylor, a little old man with oily gray hair. He could barely see, but he was a hard nut who "really knew how to skin you." Naylor lived in a room the size of a small store, and buying fur and roots was all he did. He would run his hands over a trapper's hides, feeling them up and down, and always found a reason to push the price down. "I think you got some rocks in there," he'd whine in a high voice.

Naylor paid more or less the same price every year. "You'd go in there and he would lay your roots out on an old baloney scale, and that was the end of it." No negotiating, take it or leave it.

Anglers Roost, a sporting-goods shop that has become one of the state's largest ginseng dealers, was today's version of Old Man Naylor. Fred said the store gulled diggers who dug ginseng only while hunting something else and who liked to sell their roots at the same place where they bought ammo and hunting supplies. Basically, these diggers used ginseng to pay for their hunting season.

That accurately described Tom Carte, a digger in his fifties who lived not far from Anglers Roost. Ginseng meant a lot to Carte; he and his brothers learned to dig at their uncle's mountain cabin. They would leave at daybreak carrying a bucket of biscuits and stay out until evening. You could fill trucks with the ginseng he dug, he said. Carte used the money to buy school clothes. Back then he read all he could about ginseng, and about how rare Manchurian 'sang was. (He still remembered the price paid for Asian ginseng in 1958: $1,240 per pound.) He and his brother used to pore over topographic maps to locate new ginseng patches. They knew all the ones in the nearby counties and across the state line into the Shenandoah Valley. Carte spoke of nine-prong plants with berries the size of kidney beans. But now he dug just once or twice a year, enough to cover his hunting season costs. That season he might not get into the woods at all. His time was taken up by a kitchen renovation at home and twelve-hour shifts at the mine. "I wish I had time," he told me.

After Fred and I had yakked away much of the afternoon on his porch, he took me out to dig ginseng in his woods. Most of the stems had already gone down. The tree trunks were damp and dark, against a yellowed mat of leaves. For timber-stand management, Fred stopped to cut away thick furry ropes of poison ivy from a tree trunk. I kept my eyes trained on the ground, hopeful. By now I had been out ginsenging five times, and I felt I should be able to spot the leaf cluster. Every time I thought I saw it, though, it was a tree seedling or poison ivy.

Fred wasn't having much luck either. "There was plenty here a few weeks ago," he said. The overcast sky started to spit on us.

We circled back to a poplar we had passed earlier. Fred scanned the ground again, and that's when he found it. Once the first three-prong revealed itself, others followed. In a half hour we had five roots. At that rate, a day might yield a hundred roots. Not bad for a walk in the woods, but no gold mine either.

NEAR SUNSET I DROVE out the four-lane to a racetrack outside Charleston. I looked out over the raked rows of seats and the wet oval track, and kept thinking of ginseng as a sort of gamble. What kept ginseng in the lives of people like Fred and George appeared to be a sort of trifecta. First, there was a tradition of stories that traced back through the generations to Daniel Boone's era. Then there was the prospect of just enough cash to give those stories some traction. Finally, people enjoyed the puzzle of finding an elusive plant in its native forest. But for that gamble to pay off, ginsengers had to rely on another group of people: the notorious dealers.

SIX

Courted by Traders,
and Dancing the Ginseng Polka

The shades of night were falling fast,
As o'er the muddy highway passed
A youth, who bore, across a stick,
A tin-pail, knapsack, hoe and pick!
Dig Ginseng!

. . . .

A traveler, passing by the place,
Reports, that all the vacant space
Is packed with the gigantic weed!
The youth, with unabated speed,
Digs Ginseng!

—AUTHOR UNKNOWN, *Minnesota Statesman,* May 27, 1859

The morning after my visit with Fred Hays, my hand itched where I had brushed against the poison ivy. Ginsengers call poison ivy an occupational hazard. I scratched my hand with a perverse sort of pride.

It was my last day in West Virginia, and I had an appointment with Tom Cook, a ginseng trader and owner of Anglers Roost.

Cook was impossible to reach directly by phone, but through a series of voicemail messages we arranged to meet at his Summersville store, in the state's eastern mountains. Traders were even more secretive than ginsengers. The first one I called clammed up as soon as I asked how many diggers he worked with. "I don't have any idea on that," he said. Conversations with other dealers were even shorter.

As tight-lipped as they are, ginseng dealers are also the agents of diggers' dreams, the people who turn their roots into cash. The relationship, like a quarrelsome marriage, has a long history. The names of these enterprises reveal the hodgepodge of that history: Lowe Fur and Herb, White Brothers Fur and Ginseng Company, Rainbow Recycling & Botanicals. This patchwork is a mere remnant of the trading network that grew in the century after Father Lafitau's discovery near Montreal, when the international commerce in ginseng rivaled the fur trade and attracted all kinds of agents, including John Jacob Astor, America's first multimillionaire. Astor's interest and the hopes of diggers then grew in large measure from reports of the *Empress of China,* the first U.S. ship to sail to the Far East.

When the *Empress* started out in early 1784, the new United States had no trade agreements or consulates in Asia, and hardly any in Europe. No American ship had ever ventured past Africa's southern tip. That winter was the coldest in memory, and for six weeks the ship was stalled in New York's frozen harbor, waiting for the ice to melt. Several generations of colonists had sold their ginseng to China through the British. In the 1750s, Chinese buyers had soured on Canadian ginseng when French merchants sold them roots that had been scorched from careless drying. The Canton merchants refused to buy more Canadian roots and the French trade dropped from a half million francs a year to nothing. The British colonies had rushed to fill the supply shortage, but the Revolutionary War had choked off their access to the Far East trade for nearly a decade, and it wasn't clear they could reopen it. Nevertheless, a pair of money men hired a small, copper-bottomed ship built for speed, renamed her the *Empress of China,* and outfitted her for the Far East: the $120,000 investment was roughly ten times the amount needed for a Europe-bound cargo. At the helm stood Captain John Green, a veteran of the Continental Navy.

Americans looked to Canton with great hopes. Western fascination with Chinese culture was at a peak, and its fashions swept through Europe and America; the pigtail hairstyle, porcelain, and silks. Westerners were particularly intrigued by China's long experience with herbal remedies. In considering what cargo would make the best impression, the owners of the *Empress* settled on ginseng. The ship's surgeon procured over thirty tons of American ginseng roots through a series of feverish trips up and down the mountains of Pennsylvania and Virginia, a buying spree that almost single-handedly forced up the price that season. On February 22, the *Empress* finally left New York harbor. The fact that it was George Washington's birthday was seen as a good omen.

The *Empress* was not the only vessel stocking up on ginseng that season, as it happened. It had a rival in the *Harriet,* another sloop, from Hingham, south of Boston. The *Harriet* had got the faster start and left for China in December 1783, laden with ginseng. At the Cape of Good Hope, she met up with veteran

British traders to the East Indies who were startled to learn of Yankee competitors. To squelch that challenge the British bought out the *Harriet* on the spot, paying double for her cargo. Her captain made a good bargain but lost out on the fame that would come to the *Empress.*

In August 1784, the *Empress* dropped anchor outside Canton harbor and fired off an exuberant thirteen-gun salute. Other schooners from France, Great Britain, Denmark, and Holland responded, welcoming her with return volleys. Captain Green wrote in his log book that the *Empress* "had the honour of hoisting the first Continental Flagg Ever Seen or made Euse of in those Seas."

Despite their planning, the captain and his crew had stumbled into Asia almost blind. They needed help from a French ship to navigate the rocky straits between Java and Sumatra, and they failed to bring Cantonese customs officials any of the usual courtesy gifts. Nevertheless, the *Empress* received permission to unload her cargo in a Canton harbor crammed with brightly colored ships and smaller vessels. The casks of ginseng were hauled up and stirred a commotion on the docks. One of the crew members of the *Empress* later crowed that it was "the largest quantity of ginseng ever brought to the Chinese market" at one time. A Cantonese artist captured the event with a fanciful image of the *Empress* he painted into a sweeping panorama. The Americans were assured they would be welcomed back. When the *Empress* returned home, her story of a handsome profit was published in newspapers up and down the Atlantic coast. Even before Congress could agree on a Constitution, it was moved by the *Empress's* journey to pass a resolution expressing "its peculiar satisfaction in the successful issue of this first effort of the citizens of America to establish a direct trade with China." Ginseng root became an entrepreneur's bonanza.

AMERICA'S PREMIER ENTREPRENEUR of that era, John Jacob Astor, responded eagerly. Astor had come to America during the winter of 1784. While the *Empress of China* waited in New York harbor for the ice to melt for her outbound journey, Astor waited in steerage on an inbound vessel down the coast, poised to enter the Chesapeake Bay when the ice cleared. He came from Europe with musical instruments and sheet music, and when he reached New York established himself quickly as a shrewd businessman. (Astor had left his family in Germany and visited a brother in London before continuing to Baltimore. Some sources claim that Astor bankrolled a ginseng shipment to China in 1782, but at that time he was still a teenager in Europe.) Within two years he had his own business in lower Manhattan, and advertised imported pianofortes, flutes, clarinets, and violin strings. Soon he was expanding his inventory and traveling to Montreal for new products. By the mid-1790s Astor was exploring the China trade, buying space on other merchants' ships and sending 3,300 pounds of ginseng to China along with skins of otter, beaver and fox. Some say he made fifty-five thousand dollars on another ginseng shipment before he became America's fur monopolist. Astor's coast-to-coast network of trading posts eventually created a direct Pacific link for his American Fur Company. His agents on the frontier became notorious for taking the law in their own hands and swindling Native Americans. And the fur trade, with its web of buyers and its grasp on ginseng exports, endured well into the twentieth century.

ONE OF ASTOR'S COUNTERPARTS today can be found at Anglers Roost. The outdoorsman's superstore has several outlets in West Virginia and a shopping center façade as big as a Wal-Mart. WE BUY GINSENG AND GOLDENSEAL announces a sign in front. Inside is everything the modern consumer-sportsman could ever desire. You're greeted by a standing grizzly, a wolf, a beaver, and a deer, all stuffed and poised to take your hand. Beyond them stretch racks and racks of hunting bows, rifles, and shotguns. There are aisles of sight mounts and safety vests, ammo clips and a Camo Compac (camouflage makeup kit), game bags, high-tech wading staffs with a thermometer and other weather instruments embedded on them. Here you can buy an Ugly Stik, metal traps, turkey calls and scents, and gun-cleaning rods. The fishing section has everything from rods to boats. You can buy a license to hunt or fish or dig 'sang, and afterward you can come sit and play checkers in the Lyin' Den and b.s. about what you bagged.

During my visit that morning, the owner's son offered me a cup of coffee and pointed me down a row of temporary cubicles at the front of the store, like a trailer several steps up from the vast showroom.

Inside the last door Tom Cook sat at his desk, wearing a beige shirt with forest green cuffs and a gun-butt patch on the right shoulder: the image of a sportsman—plus a pager. He had an air of informal but brisk competence. He kept moving as he spoke with me, tapping an unlit cigarette against his desk, eyes roving the retail floor behind him. Photos of children and grandchildren lined the wall alongside wry motivational proverbs. On his bulletin board hung a wild ginseng root with a wrinkled neck over four inches long, pinned to a handwritten note that states its age at fifty-eight years, a gift from the man who dug it.

"We're hillbillies," Cook said. "Some people want to call us mountaineers but hell, we're hillbillies." The next minute he told me that people from Appalachia take an eye for ginseng wherever they go, whether it's New York or Indiana. Locals in those places weren't good ginsengers until Appalachians showed them how, he said.

"The hillbilly groundhog-hunted in May and June, fished in June and July, and squirrel-hunted in October." And as summer turned to fall, he dug ginseng. A decade ago Tom Cook started positioning ginseng as recreation, "something to do between hunting seasons that gives another excuse to go out and spend time in the woods." That focus on sport fit well with his business and diverted diggers from haggling over the price. (Anglers Roost also bought diggers' black cohosh, ramps, and log moss.) When the question of price came up, Anglers Roost rested its reputation on their digital scale, accurate to 0.3 ounces on 250 pounds. Cook himself could tell you the exact weight of a grocery bag. If another dealer offered a slightly higher price per pound, Cook said, it was just bait-and-switch. "If he can steal an ounce from you he can pay an extra fifteen dollars a pound."

The owner of Anglers Roost started out in life as a ginseng digger. He learned from his father, a timbercutter and veteran of weeklong ginseng-digging expeditions with friends. At least one farm near where Cook grew up was bought with ginseng money. His father would weave back and forth across a slope, reading the landscape for signals in the terrain and timber. If he saw a walnut tree or a certain kind of rock outcropping, he would work toward it. He taught Tom by standing at the foot of a hill and directing the boy as he walked up the slope. "He'd wave me left and right like you do a damn bird dog and I'd finally step on it."

The father then showed the boy how to sell their roots to a grocer in Hillsborough. At the time, few buyers worked in that part of the state, apart from circuit-riders like F.G. Hamilton of West Augusta, Virginia, who had dealt in ginseng and furs at least since the 1940s. Hamilton, a living legend among buyers, was now in his nineties.

"Hamilton was the market. He handled most of the eastern ginseng. An awful lot of it went through him." Cook tapped a cigarette on the desk. "Hell, the son of a bitch is still buying! Can't see to sign his check. Has to use a magnifying glass. . . . But he won't quit, he won't die." Tapped the cigarette again.

When Tom Cook started buying furs back in his twenties, he also started dealing in ginseng. He rode the circuit and traveled the Blue Ridge like Hamilton. Once he bought a root from a produce-and-cider stand in Sperryville, Virginia, that weighed twenty-nine ounces. He bought roots as big as a water bucket.

For decades, Cook traced ginseng's fluctuations in detail, marking the root's dwindling tracks through the county on charts. He graphed harvests against a startling variety of factors: root weight, precipitation, temperature, and digging location, as well as indicators for deer kills, unemployment, and fur trapping. Although he conceded his graphs weren't scientific, they were meticulous. Yet they turned up no clear correlations. He had once hypothesized that ginseng harvests might rise with unemployment (figuring that people would try to compensate lost wages by hunting root) but found that when the coal companies laid off workers, the workers moved to other states with more jobs. There might be a correlation with local deer numbers: when a deer population soared, they browsed ginseng back to mere stems, making it hard for diggers to find the plants.

The one clear relationship that Cook discovered involved the quality of fur and ginseng at a particular spot. Areas that produced high-quality fur also had top-quality ginseng, he said. But for Cook, the biggest factor in what he called ginseng's "declining dig" was the dwindling network of local dealers. When a dealer passed away, casual diggers lost a familiar contact, and sometimes interest in digging. Cook's point was that ginseng goes nowhere without its human fire brigade of middlemen. Whether Fred Hays liked it or not, dealers filled gaps in the supply chain that ginsengers couldn't always cover on their own. Neither Hays nor Cook thought that ginseng would go extinct; but they both worried that the ginsenging culture—the knowledge of wild ginseng in the woods and the lore passed from one generation to the next—would disappear.

Before leaving Anglers Roost, I asked to see the storeroom where they kept the ginseng. I had a mental image of a high-security vault, trip wires and concrete. Cook hesitated.

"You got ID?" For a moment I thought he was kidding. We'd just spent an hour talking together. "If I'm not being a horse's ass . . ." I pulled out my wallet and showed him my driver's license.

As we crossed the showroom, people in the checkout lines watched us pass. I followed him behind the gun counter, a long lethal row of them, into a room lined with shelves full of more rifles, and through another cinderblock storeroom. We stopped at a fist-size padlock that he worked with two keys.

Cook was explaining that all his charts that tracked roots and their weight against unemployment and the other factors went up in flames when Anglers Roost burned down. Actually, Anglers Roost burned twice, the second time just three months before my visit. Arson. Which explains why fears about crime simmer in the back of a dealer's mind.

We were standing inside a fifteen-by-twenty-foot cinderblock shell, as fireproof as Cook could make it. It was bare except for three big brown dish barrels in the far corner and an industrial-size floor scale with a digital LED readout mounted on the wall near the door. Those three hundred-pound barrels contained about twenty thousand dollars worth of dried roots. No fancy processing, just carefully cleaned and dried. The room, if full, could probably hold an inventory worth a quarter of a million until Cook either sold the lot to a New York wholesaler or exported it himself. A state inspector would come check the ginseng and weigh it, maybe take samples. When Cook exports directly, he has to prepare the international paperwork required under the endangered species treaty and then send the roots to Philadelphia, where they exit the country, following Daniel Boone's soggy harvest by air freight to Hong Kong.

Our words echoed against the concrete walls. Cook took a lunch bag full of roots from the one open barrel and poured a handful onto the scale. The LED display read 0.12, or two ounces. He eyeballed it. "That's about thirty dollars." For the whole lunch bag full of roots, the ginsenger got a hundred and forty dollars.

ACROSS MUCH OF NORTH America that fall, roots were swarming by the millions into storerooms like the one at Anglers Roost. From north Georgia to Minnesota's west bank of the Mississippi, diggers were moved to head for the woods. Although they numbered in the thousands and together made an estimated $18 million each year (at least through legal channels), they were hard to find. There's never been a Wild Ginseng Diggers Association. Farmers who grow ginseng as a crop have associations in Wisconsin, Ontario, the Pacific Northwest, New York, West Virginia, and even Australia. Wild ginseng, however, is an underground guild, no longer on the public radar as it was in the 1800s, when Americans looked to nature for their medicinal herbs and livelihoods. One autumn not long after he published *Walden,* Henry David Thoreau made a trip to Vermont and encountered people collecting ginseng and cohosh. He wrote of the mountain near Brattleboro "wearing a misty cap each morning," and of women who made their "pin money," or spending money, by collecting and selling ginseng, snakeroot (*Aristolochia serpentaria,* used as a tonic) and goldenthread (*Coptis trifolia,* a bitter root used in New England to treat children with thrush).

Over a hundred years later, William Lass, like Thoreau, was on the lookout for evidence of how people made a living from nature. In the 1960s Lass, a history professor at Mankato State College, about an hour and a half outside Minneapolis, stumbled onto signs of an outbreak of ginseng fever. Lass, who habitually kept an eye peeled for objects that could make history real for his students, one day found himself in the Mankato office of Ohsman & Sons, which bought furs from trappers. He asked the manager, Herman Ohsman, if he could borrow some pelts to convince his students that Minnesota had once supported a fur industry. In the back room of the small shop, they talked about furs and about the ginseng that Ohsman had bought from trappers at least since the 1930s. Ohsman's father had started the business in Iowa. It had branches in Mankato, Illinois, and New York, and shipped furs and roots to Europe and the Far East.

Not long after that, Lass was researching the state's history with the Dakota and Winnebago when he came across several yellowed newspaper articles that pointed him to the remarkable incident of Minnesota's Ginseng Rush. Intrigued by the first few articles, he delved further. From old dailies and weeklies published in towns around the Big Woods region, he pieced together the story of an episode overlooked in official histories.

IN THE 1850s MANKATO was a steamboat landing on the Minnesota River. From the edge of town, Minnesota's Big Woods stretched north over a hundred miles to St. Cloud, on the Mississippi, and eastward to Rush City on the St. Croix River. The thick forest held mostly basswood, sugar maple, elm, and oak in the north; between the two rivers in the south, the woods were mainly oaks and conifers. Minnesota was still being settled, and the forest remained largely unfamiliar to newcomers who staked their claims in towns or on farmland. Then a major land trust went bust, and the state's economy tumbled into depression.

In the fall of 1858 three men arrived at the edges of the Big Woods looking for roots. On the forest's southern edge in St.

Peter, Col. B.F. Pratt, reportedly from Virginia, paid locals to scout the area for ginseng. Pratt was understood to have a contract "with some heavy root doctor in the east." At the same time in Wayzata, near Minneapolis, the Chilton brothers from Iowa started buying and drying ginseng. Not much later, shipments of the root started arriving at the receiving dock of a Philadelphia exporter. The Minnesota point-of-origin label was smeared past legibility, apparently by someone who wanted to keep a discovery to himself. In May of 1859 the newspapers reported the previous fall's ginseng harvest—about $10,000 (or $210,000 in 2004 dollars). The secret was out. Almost immediately, scores of men were digging root in the woods near St. Peter. By the end of the month diggers claimed earnings of up to five dollars a day (over a hundred dollars a day now). One of the Chilton brothers showed up from Virginia with a lot of money, the *Minnesota Statesman* reported. A new ginseng-drying facility on Lake Washington was touted as a boon to the unemployed people in the area, "as these diggings will bring the gold more certainly than those at Pike's peak" (a reference to a Colorado gold strike that soon fizzled).

Meanwhile at the north edge of the Big Woods more mysterious Virginians showed up. One evening in Rockford, two men asked if ginseng grew nearby. The next morning locals brought a root to the older of the two, a well-dressed gentleman named Robert Blaine. Blaine promptly offered good money to anyone who brought him more roots like that one.

Handbills appeared on roadsides and street corners in towns throughout the area, offering a high price for ginseng. Wagonloads of people and tools came from Minneapolis, headed into the Big Woods for ginseng expeditions. Groups appeared from Wisconsin and beyond. The rush was on.

If you had stood in the woods and squinted, the scene of men combing the underbrush on their knees probably would have resembled what was happening just then in the forests of northeastern China. In Minnesota, as in Manchuria, diggers struck into the forest in early morning with a sack and a ginseng hoe, and worked until they filled the sack or daylight faded. Daily yields of ten to twenty pounds were common, with some up to fifty pounds. As in Manchuria, some Minnesota diggers got hopelessly lost in the woods. Others complained of being exploited by dealers who paid them eight cents a pound and then turned around and sold the root for nine or ten times as much (after washing and drying).

By early June, the *Daily Pioneer and Democrat* reported that towns were emptied of able bodies and the forest was full of them:

> bar-rooms are abandoned; eucher and draw-poker have lost their facination [sic]; even fishing, ducking, politics and re-ligion are not now displayed as peculiar fortes; but old and young, the patrician and the plebian, the prudent and the desolate are all agog with—'Ginseng.'

Everybody in St. Peter who could not otherwise make three dollars a day was out in the woods digging sang. The *Red Wing Sentinel* ran a banner headline: GINSENG FEVER. In Chatfield, some residents made roughly a hundred dollars in a week of digging. Minnesota was catapulted to the front of ginseng-producing states.

People around the Big Woods saw ginseng as a godsend. The *Minnesota Statesman* published poems about the root. The town of Mankato threw a ball in its honor. An announcement for that celebration said the dance would distract diggers from the "musquito bite or toil of delving for the bulbous root, whilst 'tripping the light fantastic toe.'" You can imagine the scene in the town's Union Hall, a clapboard structure on the main street near the river: the summer twilight lasting longest then, and the dance numbers following a familiar sequence, up to the newly composed Ginseng Polka.

The music faded quickly. By late June the boomlet had stalled. Roots had flooded into exporters' warehouses back east faster than the market could absorb them. The price slumped. Still, the fling had helped many people make their mortgage payments and buy groceries, and for three years the state shipped more than half of the total U.S. ginseng harvest. Sometimes twenty-five tons left St. Paul in a single week. Although it never struck again with quite the same intensity, Minnesota's ginseng fever simmered into the early 1860s. By 1861, the main diggers were the Sioux and Winnebago along the Minnesota River at the western frontier, along with smaller-scale diggers like farm boys and housewives who sold it for spending money.

In 1865 the Minnesota legislature passed "An Act to preserve and protect the growth of Ginseng." It was probably the first regulation that restricted American ginseng hunting to a season, which the law set as May 1 to August 1. Digging at other times became a misdemeanor subject to a fine of up to a hundred dollars. The law aimed to reassure the moneymen back east that they could depend on a regular supply of quality Minnesota roots in the future. Yet within thirty years the root was just about dug out of Minnesota. By the 1890s, old-timers of the '59 rush had grown nostalgic. Articles in the *Faribault Republican* and the *Wright County Republican* recalled the old days when ginseng saved Minnesota.

"What made the 1859 episode unique," Lass told me, "was that it came when the Minnesota economy had crashed. So you found many people out in the woods collecting it who otherwise wouldn't have been there." In the article Lass wrote about the Minnesota Ginseng Rush for the state's history journal, he had called it a "legendary" interlude that helped pioneers through perilous times.

"Are you aware," he added slowly, "that the United States government at one point encouraged the production of ginseng?"

Near the end of our conversation, Dr. Lass mentioned that just a week before, he had spoken with someone who knew someone who reportedly had "gone out and gathered the wild root," he said, the last word rhyming with *soot*. He offered to put me in contact with that individual.

While there may be a few diggers left in Mankato, the town's last trader was gone. Herman Ohsman lived just long enough to see the fur market vanish and ginseng decline. A few years after he died, the company closed its Mankato office. Today his great-nephew Mike Ohsman owns the family-owned company, still based in Cedar Rapids, Iowa. They got out of ginseng when supply of the wild root dwindled and the price fluctuated too much. When it became an endangered species, the mounting paperwork ended ginseng as an enterprise for Ohsman. He said they weren't in the business of counting rings on the neck of each root.

BOOMS LIKE THE ONE in Minnesota explain why ginseng pops up in songs, verse, and stories. There are other plants that inspire celebratory festivals and statues: corn has the Corn Palace in South Dakota and a city fountain in Peru's Sacred Valley of the Incas. Potato festivals are all over the place. There's even a festival for ramps—a kind of wild leek—in West Virginia. But ginseng leaves a wistful note that's unique. Its allure and illicit undertones are captured in "Ginseng," a poem by Indianapolis reporter Jared Carter:

> Even now,
> He explained, men dig it up, ruin
> Whole stands, steal it from farmers.
> But all of them together—hunters,
> Thieves, those who keep the old ways—
> Pass it from hand to hand along
> A chain of those who know exactly
> Where it is going, what it is worth—
> Until eventually it arrives
> On the other side of the world.
> Where it is ground into dust
> And mixed into potions they say
> Can make an old man young again.

There's the mystery of "potions" and an elixir of youth, elements that don't quite suit a plant of progress. Maybe ginseng was a plant of a backward-looking regime. That's the tone of "Ginseng Sullivan," a song about a long-haired, aging worrywart who yearns to leave his shack in the north Georgia hills and return to the Mississippi Delta. But he frets that he won't ever be able to get home because his ticket depends on how much he gets for the next summer's roots. The song, by old-time musician Norman Blake, is a crippling blend of fear, hope, and longing.

In America, these hopes seem to stem from the stories brought back by the *Empress of China.* When she came back to New York with a trove of tea, silks, and china, the *Empress* paid a substantial twenty-five percent profit to her investors. She also spawned her share of regrets: when she returned to China the following year, European crews regarded her as a competitor. In Canton, Samuel Shaw, the ship's business agent, would find Captain Green spreading scurrilous rumors about him. Shaw would have challenged Green to a duel, except for the fact that Chinese law regarded dueling as simply murder, for which the punishment was strangulation. The *Empress* herself was later sold and renamed; she sank in Dublin Bay in 1791. None of this, however, dimmed the tales of the ship's triumph that would hearten Astor and other ginseng traders deeper in the countryside.

TODAY SOME OF THE largest traders are in Wisconsin, including Hsu's Ginseng, the country's top dealer in cultivated ginseng and a principal buyer of wild roots as well. The company began in the 1970s and by 1994 was handling a third of all American ginseng exports to Asia. When I called, the marketing director said they had just shipped a container load to Asia and expected to send another later that fall. He said I could visit in October when founder Paul Hsu would be back from China, where he was growing his franchise.

So continues the lure of roots and cash. I caught up with William Lass's ginseng-digger friend in Minnesota. George Schmeling grew up on the west bank of the Mississippi, two hours downstream from Red Wing, and learned how to hunt ginseng from his father on the rocky bluffs above the river. Then he moved away, took a job farther north, and forgot about shang for twenty years. Eventually Schmeling moved back to Mankato. One fall he went out in the woods with his brother-in-law, back to the bluffs where he grew up, and the memory came back. Schmeling found ginseng there, and in other woods nearby, big roots in ravines off the Minnesota River and under elms. He found ginseng not just on northern slopes but on south-, east-, and west-facing slopes, too. He found it under oaks near his sister-in-law's place to the northwest, where nobody expected to find it anymore. The roots were like old coins discovered in a dusty family heirloom.

Now Schmeling thinks a lot about where the plant grows and what makes the root's wrinkled neck. He has sold roots to the same dealer for thirteen years, getting $425 per pound, not far off the peak of $525 a few years before. He finds himself walking the woods near the road for hours in the early morning after working the night shift of his maintenance job, scanning the forest understory for the telltale leaf. Late September is the best time, he said, when the leaf turns that unique shade of yellow.

My mind conjured the image of thousands of wild ginsengers stretched from northern Georgia to eastern Minnesota, united in their solitary moments by an ineffable bond, a shared focus. People like George Schmeling, leaving the night shift and wandering alone for miles, were keeping an eye open for the plant that gives meaning and music to those long, lonely walks in the woods.

SEVEN

Traders Again

History and science have their romances as vivid
and as fascinating as any in the realms of fiction. No story
ever told has surpassed in interest the history of this
mysterious plant Ginseng . . .

—A. R. HARDING,
Ginseng and Other Medicinal Plants, 1936 edition

On a brisk autumn day, David Law, the country's leading exporter of wild ginseng, welcomed me into his home office in Manhattan. The ginsengers I had spoken with regarded wholesalers like Law as snakeheads in the roots' middle passage to Asia, even worse than the roadside retail buyers. The big brokers hustled root to warehouses and shipped it out to Asia (most of it landed within a few hundred miles of the port that had welcomed the *Empress of China*). Park rangers said that the big dealers manipulated the ginseng market the way that OPEC rigged the oil market. They could raise the price they paid and send thousands of diggers out beating the woods for root. Just as suddenly, they could drop the price, forcing ginsengers to sell their roots cheap or hold tight until the next year. The consensus was that all dealers would, like Old Man Naylor, squint at your root and screw you out of your fair share.

Dealers held a different view, of course. For example, Ray Bowkley, a top North Carolina dealer, painted himself as a long-suffering entrepreneur who had to reckon with a formidable series of obstacles to help producers get their product to market. "People like me are squishy middlemen," Bowkley said. "The interesting part of this business is out in the woods." In his twenty-five years of dealing ginseng (he started right out of high school), Bowkley had weathered dramatic shifts in the industry. At first, he sold his ginseng to the New York furriers like everybody else; when the fur business died, he had to cobble together a new series of contacts. Now that Chinese importer-exporters had bypassed the old New York brokers, the world had become a smaller place. Not a cozy place, mind you. More like a cramped family home. Bowkley got competition from the Cherokee reservation, where dealers could pay a slightly higher price because they weren't subject to state laws and taxes. Then Korean buyers would sweep through during the season and pay very high prices for small amounts of fresh ginseng that suited their niche market. That left ginsengers with unrealistically high expectations, and Bowkley had to talk sense back into them. There's also the bureaucracy. Bowkley's hometown was just five miles from the Tennessee line, but because Tennessee's ginseng season starts a month before North Carolina's, Bowkley lost a month to buyers a few miles away. State inspectors came to his office and riffled his paperwork (he needed a certificate from the state's Department of Agriculture before his ginseng could leave North Carolina), and extension agents like Dave Cooke and

Bob Beyfuss confused diggers with new ideas about simulated-wild ginseng and getting more money for their roots. To Bowkley, that kind of talk sounded like bureaucrats desperate to steer farmers away from a dying tobacco industry and its government subsidies, even if that meant more risk to the farmers. "To be cynical, which I often am," Bowkley said, "that gets the monkey off the government agent's back, onto the farmer's."

Dealers further up the market chain shared Bowkley's penchant for a low profile. When David Law greeted me at the door of an unassuming brick house on Manhattan's Lexington Avenue, he was wearing a plain white T-shirt, black shorts, and low white sport socks with sneakers. He had a few gray hairs, but his rounded face looked youngish and his bursts of laughter reminded me of Ed Wynne floating around the room in *Mary Poppins*. David Law did not put on airs.

"Right now," he said. "The digging is going on right now."

He invited me down to his basement office. The first floor was dimly lit by a bulb in the large aquarium near the front door. As we descended to the basement the first thing I saw at the foot of the steps was a scale with a large box on it, a cube two feet on each side, postmarked from rural Virginia. Then I noticed, crammed along the walls, fourteen brown dish barrels full of root—1,400 pounds, or over a half a million dollars worth, by my arithmetic. Like the barrels in Anglers Roost, these resembled huge ice-cream containers. There were so many they obscured the fluorescent-lit desk at the back, which was silted with paper and notebooks. Off to the side was a large flat-screen computer monitor and a fine stereo system, the only two things in the room that looked new. Law rolled his black desk chair over for me and he sat in a smaller one. While we talked, he leaned back often, lit a cigarette, fished out a checkbook, looked over figures in his notebook, shushed the dachshund barking outside the back door.

A native of Guangzhou (formerly Canton), Law grew up in Hong Kong. After more than a quarter of a century dealing in American ginseng, he called it "a dead-end business." Farmers who grew cultivated ginseng were getting hammered by the high costs of pesticides, and wild-ginseng diggers were running out of supply. When Law started buying wild ginseng in America in the mid-1970s, the ginseng graders' guild in Hong Kong would hold an auction almost every week where he would sell eight or ten hundred-pound drums. Sometimes twenty drums, or two thousand pounds a week. Now, even as U.S. demand for ginseng products was climbing, the dwindling wild ginseng harvests and a shift in Asian demand were making it hard to scare up three auctions a year.

Nonetheless, every fall Law takes a four- to six-week driving trip through the heart of wild ginseng country to buy his annual inventory. Law's first expedition began in April 1976, and remained clear in his mind: he started at Williamsport, Pennsylvania, and wended south through West Virginia, Virginia, and North Carolina, then skirted west through Tennessee, Kentucky, Missouri, Iowa, and Wisconsin. It lasted over two months and involved a tremendous amount of salesmanship for the twenty-something Cantonese chemist. He had to prove his trustworthiness to old-timers like F.G. Hamilton, who lived in the mountains west of the Shenandoah Valley.

Law recalls driving the backroads of Virginia with a map on

his passenger's seat, looking for Mr. Hamilton's place. He had never met the man, but he knew that Hamilton was one of the biggest buyers in Appalachia, handling over ten thousand pounds of wild ginseng every year. The elderly bachelor lived like a hermit in an old house with a cast-iron woodstove. There was an awkward moment at the door, and then Law was invited in. He still recalls seeing the woodstove and being surprised by its rustic dimensions. He was a long way from Hong Kong.

GINSENG DEALERS HAVE LOST ground in many ways, Law told me. But they've also gotten stronger. In the early days, his suppliers dealt in everything from furs to sporting goods to groceries. "A grocery store," he'd say, "or sometimes gasoline! A gasoline station." He might cover West Virginia in a day, chartering a puddle-jumper to touch down at five or six spots in the state, and then fly back to Charleston. Or he might drive the route instead.

Law had a fascinating, off-the-cuff way of talking. Sometimes he seemed to be trying out answers to hear how they sounded or to see how I would react. Throughout our conversation he revised himself.

He grabbed a handwritten notebook. "Last year we bought about . . ." He flipped through its pages. "I shipped out fourteen thousand [pounds] altogether. You see?" He turned another page. "Everything is on record."

He didn't set out to be America's top wild-ginseng dealer. He came to the United States as a young man in the early 1970s to study at the University of South Carolina. He majored in chemistry and was interested in modern industry, not herbal medicine. After graduation he took a job with DuPont and spent several years moving up the ladder there. Then he went to Allied Chemical, conducting fuel tests at JFK airport: kerosene, PT-4, and others. Not an exciting job, but it got him to New York, where his fiancée lived. At the airfield every day, Law would check fuel quality by igniting it in a test area near the runways. He would test the water content and gauge the carbon content by how the fuel burned. Sometimes the smoke from the fuel tests billowed up ten stories high, but they could put it out in a few seconds. When he got home at night, his clothes stank of jet fuel.

"I wasn't really happy working in the airport," Law said. "It was so damn boring."

So when an acquaintance from Hong Kong called in the mid-1970s and asked him to drop what he was doing and join their ginseng business, Law thought about it. At that time, the New York furriers still had a lock on the ginseng trade. They handled things old school, making deals by mail or phone call. Law didn't know anything about ginseng, but it looked better than setting fires at the airport.

When he started dealing in the root, it was exciting. "On a good day I bought eight thousand pounds," he said. "In one day. Wild ginseng."

Law was one of the first to use a telex machine to take orders from Hong Kong. (Some of his clients still prefer telex because you can automatically confirm receipt of a telex in a way that's not always possible with a fax.) In 1975, he got a telex from Hong Kong: "David, go out and clean up the market."

"So I *did* clean up the market. All I had to do was walk along Twenty-ninth Street towards the West Side, where the first

World Trade Center building was," he said. "There were three stores that sold ginseng. You'd go in there in the morning before the other guy got up."

He would go into the first shop and ask how much they had. Five thousand pounds? He punched in calculations on an invisible calculator. Okay. Then he'd stop for a cup of coffee, walk to the next store. Buy their whole inventory.

Within a few hours, Law had bought eight thousand pounds. Back then you could deal on that kind of a scale. But he had never paid attention back in Hong Kong when his father had dealt in ginseng ("I was the black sheep"), so David still had a lot to learn. Sometimes he didn't time his purchases well, or he messed up a shipment. He flapped his lips with a finger, mocking the crazy missteps of his youth.

"You make stupid mistakes, right? You may end up losing thousands of dollars, but because of the up market, you may get through."

He had competitors but not enemies, he said. Sure, he knew Wisconsin mogul Paul Hsu. "Competitor with me, yeah," Law said. "I've known him since seventy-six! No, no, no. I think 1978, he opened up his store. Seventy-eight."

"So it's a small community—"

"No!" he said. "At that time there were quite a lot of ginseng buyers. There were quite a lot more. You'd be surprised! A lot of them don't exist anymore." In the Seventies he could buy ginseng from over two hundred dealers, but that pool has shrunk to about fifty. So in the decades that U.S. appetite for ginseng has grown, the number of dealers has dwindled. America seems to be shifting from a ginseng supplier to a consumer, like China.

U.S. consumers buy Asian ginseng products as often as American ginseng, with roots imported from China, South Korea, and Hong Kong. In the first quarter of 2004, for example, the United States imported nearly 157,000 kilograms of ginseng from Asia—more roots by weight than it exported. But cultivated American ginseng gets a better price, so there's no move to grow the Asian variety here.

Now, after a boom in the 1990s, the market for cultivated ginseng was so low that it almost made Law feel guilty. He saw the rising costs of agrochemicals and the shrinking price for cultivated ginseng squeeze many farmers out of business. He blamed the bureaucracy. The EPA had banned certain fungicides, for example, that Canadians could still use, so Canadian farmers were getting yields nearly double what Wisconsin growers could get. Law told me about one farmer whom he had known for twenty years. The farmer had five acres of ginseng. With fungicides, fertilizers, and labor, it cost him $40,000 to grow an acre of ginseng, so he had invested $200,000 in his crop, most of it with a bank loan. But the wet weather had pummeled the roots that year and his total harvest amounted to two hundred pounds—a fraction of the normal yield. The farmer was on the brink of bankruptcy and furious over his debts. He grumbled about filing a lawsuit against the agrochemical company.

"He was crying when he took my check," Law said. "Two and a half drums, that's it."

They had stood at the edge of the field, the wooden shade trellises uncovered, the rows of earth brown after the harvest. They looked at the drums and then at each other. Then they loaded the drums into the back of Law's rented pickup.

"We didn't know what to say," Law said. "It's been twenty years that I've been buying his ginseng, and this shit thing happens. This year will be his last year.

"It's tough to make deals like that," he admitted. "You walk in there, the farmer asks for a price, you don't want to negotiate. And even though you know you're paying him a couple of dollars more, or ten dollars more, it's just . . . so sad. The amount is so small, you know?"

Law fished around in the papers on his desk and came up with the checkbook containing the carbon of last year's check. He studied it. He had rounded the amount upward. "Two thousand dollars I paid him. A whole year's harvest," he said quietly. "That's *miserable,* isn't it?"

LAW HAD TWO MAIN complaints about the ginseng business now. The first was problems with China. When he said "problems," I thought he meant the steep tariff that China had long imposed on ginseng imports, tariffs that were expected to shrink now that China was joining the World Trade Organization.

"The problem is not the tariff," Law said. "The problem is corruption."

Say the whole world needs just a hundred shoes. If world production stays at a hundred shoes, everybody makes a little money. The problem was that China was producing a thousand shoes.

"Why are you producing a thousand shoes?" he asked.

"Maybe once the production within China stabilizes—" I said.

"No, China is not going to be stabilizing," Law insisted.

"China is going to be increasing, because at that price they still make money. Not a lot, but they still make money. Just like the Canadians."

That was his second complaint: Canada was growing way too much cultivated ginseng, having passed U.S. production years ago. (Canada has outlawed the collection of wild ginseng.) Canadian farmers grew more than ten times as much ginseng as they used to—over five million pounds a year. And U.S. growers had only themselves to blame, Law said. He traced it back to a convention in Guelph, Canada, in the mid-1980s that created too much interest in ginseng. That convention alone, Law said, converted over two hundred Canadian farmers to ginseng growers. Wisconsin people had sold them their seed.

"That damn convention in Canada! That was the biggest mistake they ever made. Because at that time, the Canadian farmer was feeling the pain. The tobacco farmers were feeling the pain, and now this, a new relief." The Canadian tobacco farmers had land, they had capital, they had equipment. Turning them into ginseng competitors was asking for trouble.

"It was the biggest mistake," he repeated, shaking his head. "A couple of wiseguys sold them ginseng seeds. I remember I was in the parking lot. I read this: 'A hundred dollars a pound. Ginseng seed. Cash. Ten thousand dollars, buy a bag of ginseng seed.' I saw that ad with my own eyes! I know the buyers and the sellers, too." It was as if he was reliving a drug deal gone bad, one that he couldn't stop.

"It's a bad trade, I tell you," he said finally. "I'll be surprised if I survive the whole—" He searched for the right word. "—end tail of the damn business!"

I couldn't tell how much was smokescreen and how much was world-weariness. He seemed capable of both.

LEAVING LAW'S OFFICE, I waited for the uptown Six train in the Astor Place subway station. Standing by the tracks, I stared at a curious motif in the Beaux Arts tiles on the wall: *Astor* was spelled in green, and at intervals large rodents gnawed on a plant. I stepped closer and realized, from the flat tail, that the rodent was actually a beaver. The walls commemorated that humble source of John Jacob Astor's wealth and power. I walked to the other end of the platform. All the tiles had the same beaver. I didn't see any tiles commemorating the plant that was another source of Astor's wealth.

On the train I recalled one of the root's earliest hucksters, William Byrd, a Virginia aristocrat and gambler. As a law student in London in the early 1700s, Byrd stirred up interest in ginseng at meetings of the Royal Society, calling it a "king of plants" that helped all kinds of illnesses. He wrote letters that claimed ginseng "gives an uncommon Warmth and Vigor to the Blood, and frisks the Spirit, beyond any other cordial." Byrd waxed as pithy as a Burma Shave ad writer: "It will even make Old Age amicable, by rendering it lively, chearful [sic], and good-humour'd." (This same William Byrd published an anonymous tract on the health benefits of tobacco for preventing the plague.) Byrd stopped short of claiming that the root was an aphrodisiac. He had a healthy appreciation for the absurd. Ginseng, he cautioned, grew "as sparingly as Truth & Public Spirit."

Once the trade in American ginseng to China got under way, European shipping agents tried to finagle samples of Asian ginseng so they could gauge the competition. Business heated up, and when American traders entered the fray they tried to circumvent the Cantonese monopoly. They nosed around in shops near the Canton harbor, looking for shopkeepers willing to buy ginseng outside the monopoly. This pushed the Co Hong merchants' guild closer to the English, who followed the rules. In response, the Americans cut their shipping rates to undercut the British on tea and other items.

The ginseng business continued to hone people's ability to skirt the bureaucracy and stiff their competitors. In 1947, Syl Yunker was a teenaged U.S. army recruit in Korea, where he fell in with a Virginian whom the Koreans had hired to rebuild their government agricultural monopoly. The agency focused on tobacco and ginseng. Yunker had never dug ginseng back in Kentucky. His first glimpse of the plant was a patch in Korea, surrounded by guard towers, each armed with a mounted machine gun. He quickly learned that ginseng was money.

For the first year that Yunker was there, the Koreans shipped their ginseng to Shanghai and Tenzen. Then China's Communists exiled the Nationalists to Taiwan, and Mao Zedong closed the mainland ports to foreign trade. (Mao also briefly discouraged use of ginseng as part of an early birth-control policy.) But even Mao couldn't change the market.

"When Mao closed the ports, we just took it all down to Hong Kong," Yunker told me. "There was no hitch at all in price or volume." The move did, however, give a de facto monopoly in American ginseng to merchants in Hong Kong. For decades, all the American ginseng coming to China funneled through Hong Kong, then officially disappeared.

In 1966, the Hong Kong government opened an office to monitor species under CITES, an international treaty that regulates trade in endangered plants and animals. American ginseng was added to the list of plants and animals that they observed, and under the Hong Kong agency for agriculture and forestry, they started tracking the wild root. Merely processing the fifteen thousand import/export permits a year was a tremendous job for a staff of fifteen.

The challenge, in other words, remained formidable. Hong Kong returned to China's control in 1997, while retaining a degree of semi-autonomy summed up in the slogan "One country, two systems." China was embracing international trade more directly. The channels that governed how ginseng flowed through the world were shifting. Sometimes it seemed the only way to gauge that river of wild roots was to leave the world of legal stamps and permits behind and wade into darker waters.

EIGHT

Outlaws on the Road to Nowhere

*I searched two seasons and found a single root of the
wild mountain ginseng, which is esteemed so rare and precious
a thing by the doctors that the Lady Om and I could have lived
a year in comfort from the sale of our one root. But in the selling
of it I was apprehended, the root confiscated, and I was
better beaten and longer planked than ordinarily.*

—JACK LONDON, *The Jacket*, 1914

There was a moment one evening in the Great Smokies national park when I paused—the foliage was brushed with late sunlight and shadows. I was walking behind a park ranger, noticing the pistol on his right hip, following him into the glare of the low sun. Light flooded around every upright trunk and shone through the yellowing understory ahead of us. He stopped and turned his head, and in that second I wasn't sure if we were after a plant or a criminal. We continued forward, then stopped again, scanning the ground.

GINSENG IS NO STRANGER to crime. Sometimes it's the alibi, occasionally the motive, often a victim. Long before

Father Lafitau had the eureka moment that turned American ginseng into a commercial hot potato, poachers in China were pilfering Asian ginseng from the emperor's forests. International trade merely opened new horizons for smuggling and criminality. Wild ginseng's black markets now span at least three continents. In early 2000, TRAFFIC International covertly sent investigators into medicinal shops across Europe. Nearly a third of the 150 shops they visited—in France, Belgium, Germany, the Netherlands, and the United Kingdom—sold ginseng illegally, along with other rare species. When the authorities were tipped off, it sparked arrests and seizures of contraband in all five countries. In one instance, a dragnet in Brussels caught three Asian groceries and snared a pile of ginseng roots as well as plasters of tiger bone.

Siberia holds the world's last significant patches of wild Asian ginseng (not to be confused with so-called "Siberian ginseng," which is *Eleutherococcus senticosus* and not ginseng at all). In black markets near Vladivostok, the root is worth up to $25,000 per kilogram (about $11,364 per pound). Every year roughly $50 million of wild Asian ginseng is smuggled into northern China through sleepy border towns such as Markovo and Poltavka, or in boats from the tiny ports of Olga and Terney. A covert survey found that although each village had only two to three smugglers, many accomplices stood behind them. In Chuguyevka, for example, over half the town's workforce made money from illegal ginseng. When Russian investigators infiltrated a crime ring in the 1990s they found traffickers in ginseng, tiger skins, and bear parts.

As wild Asian ginseng trickles into China through its northern border, wild American ginseng floods in from the south. Hong Kong newspapers occasionally cite increases in ginseng smuggling to the mainland, or report ginseng robberies on the island. In one case, a Hong Kong decorator wearing a doctor's white lab coat lifted roots from a clinic (along with birds' nests, sharks fin, and dried scallops). He was caught hiding in a nearby restroom with over $100,000 worth of medicinals and seafood. In South Korea, a man was jailed and fined over $21,000 for stealing and eating someone else's 150-year-old ginseng root.

Ginseng has a criminal past in America as well. In the 1890s New York newspapers described a racket involving ginsengers in the Great Smoky Mountains. Complaints from Chinese ginseng merchants in San Francisco and Hong Kong pointed to a scam in which roots had been hollowed out and refilled with lead to boost their weight. For the most part, though, ginseng crimes in the United States tend to be more local. The threat that worries growers most is poaching by neighbors like Chicken Charley. Everyone from New England down fears for their 'sang being stolen, but some regions are more secretive than others. Bob Beyfuss thinks that ginseng poaching is less common in New York than in the South. He knows that in southern parks like the Great Smoky Mountains, the 'sang gets hammered. Beyfuss argues that the best insurance against theft is to tell all your neighbors that you're growing ginseng: Post signs, put up fences, let everyone know. That way, you establish your claim and poachers can't say they didn't know the land was private.

Nobody in Appalachia would advise that approach. If you tell your neighbors in western North Carolina that you're growing 'sang, you might as well put a bull's-eye on it. Your ginseng

will disappear. Appalachian growers, says agricultural agent Jeanine
Davis, have excellent reasons for secrecy. Davis's home district
in western North Carolina is a prime spot for finding ginseng's
outlaw element.

Davis is a tall and generously built woman with an outsize
laugh and no Southern accent. Before coming to North Carolina as an agricultural agent, she lived in Illinois, Kentucky,
New York, suburban Philadelphia, and the Pacific Northwest.
No place, however, prepared her for her new post.

"Western North Carolina is almost like a different country at
times," she says. "When I first started in this industry, I was so
incredibly naive."

When Davis came to work at the western Carolina agricultural experiment station near Asheville, she was the first female
faculty member in that part of the state, and she was very preg-
nant. Davis's predecessor had managed a ginseng program, so
one of the first things Davis did was plan a conference on ginseng. She believed, like Beyfuss, that raising awareness would
help solve a problem like poaching. (That belief is characteris-
tic of extension workers.)

When locals heard about her plans for a ginseng conference,
many were intrigued but hid their faces when they came by to
ask about it. Nobody wanted the information mailed to their
homes. Davis was struck by how far people went to distance
themselves from her. The paranoia was phenomenal. People
didn't want their families or neighbors to know they knew anything about ginseng. One man quietly asked Davis to send ginseng pamphlets to an address two counties away from where he
lived. He didn't want his mailman to know he *thought* about

ginseng. When Davis took photos of his ginseng patch later for educational presentations, she had to crop them to delete any landscape feature that suggested its location.

In the North Carolina hills, ginseng theft was sport and the root belonged to the bold. Victims had no recourse. Diggers warned Davis that the police weren't to be trusted to track down root poachers.

Davis considered that and reasoned that the problem was a lack of understanding by enforcement officials. So she called the district attorney and explained that ginseng wasn't just a wild plant, it was a valuable crop as worthy of legal protection as a farmer's herd of dairy cows. She pointed out the relevant laws under which ginseng theft was a felony, as long as the landowner had installed a fence. The D.A. was onboard with Davis's plan to educate police officers about the plant's value when local growers found out and begged her to stop. There were too many sheriffs and deputies related to poachers, they insisted.

"It was a real education for me," Davis says. She describes her first years in North Carolina as a time when she learned "the whole culture around ginseng." She discovered the inventions that people used to discourage poachers: one person parked a small trailer on their land and left a radio playing inside and laundry on a clothesline, all to create the illusion that someone was home. Others fashioned boxes to resemble surveillance cameras. Some employed a big dog or a shotgun that could be fired once in a while to scare off intruders. Some invested in wireless technologies, gate sensors that signaled when a gate chain is cut, or alarm systems that rang at your house or flashed lights or set off bells.

"Going out in the forest to collect these wild plants is like fishing, hunting, playing golf for some people," Davis says. "It's part of what we do here."

People in western Carolina regard ginseng as a God-given right. If you find ginseng growing on somebody's property you might ask their permission, but if nobody owns the land you don't ask. Russ McLean has practiced law there for over twenty-five years, and he has seen outsiders buy up mountain land for retirement homes. It's hard to know who owns a hillside now, he says, and it's even harder to ask absentee landowners for their permission to dig. Same with the national park. But now that the federal government has realized that ginseng is valuable—"that this natural resource that they have been graced with in the national parks is a product which a lot of people tend to dig and sell," as McLean puts it—park officials want to keep it to themselves. McLean thinks that park rangers have become overzealous in punishing people who are, after all, just practicing their way of life, a tradition older than any national park.

THE GREAT SMOKY MOUNTAINS National Park straddles the North Carolina–Tennessee line and some of the highest peaks in the Southern Appalachians. Its spectacular views, old-growth forests, and varied hiking trails make it the country's most visited national park. The Twin Creeks Natural Resource Center on the park's northern edge is a secluded log cabin in the Tennessee woods. The common room has government-issue paneling and metal chairs, with a duty board and names written in Magic Marker. A white butterfly net leans against one wall.

This is where park botanist Janet Rock works, and where she fights crime.

The Twin Creeks center houses a forensics lab for plants that appear headed for extinction. 'Sang often ends up on ice downstairs, in the botanical equivalent of a morgue. That's where rangers bring the plants confiscated from poachers. It gets logged in as evidence in criminal proceedings, like heroin in a drug trial, and entrusted to Rock. To avoid tempting anyone, she keeps the ginseng stored out of sight.

Rock wears forest-green slacks and a gray-green shirt with a Park Service shoulder patch. Her hair is cut to her collarbone, and she has deep blue eyes. She fell in love with the Smokies when she first came here for college and has been in these mountains for over twenty years, but people still don't consider her local.

Rock got drawn into the outlaw side of ginseng in 1991, when she began to monitor rare plants full-time. Around that time Twin Creeks began to receive roots that rangers had seized from poachers. Rock and her supervisor realized these seizures were a way to gauge harvest levels and the ginseng population's overall health. And they grew alarmed by the steep rise in the amount of ginseng harvested illegally. Then in 1993 rangers at Deep Creek, on the park's southern edge, made two big arrests back-to-back. In both cases, groups of men had hiked deep into the park on extended poaching expeditions. Each group came out with around fourteen pounds of root. That was a quantum leap over previous ginseng poachers, who usually had a few dozen roots on them.

Around that time, Rock and another colleague briefed the

park's law enforcement team on plant populations that were under threat. Rock showed them graphs of ginseng harvest levels
and plant demographics. She told them a similar pattern was
emerging for black cohosh, ramps, log moss, and even butter-
cups, which were also poached from the park. If the current
harvest rates continued, she said, all those plants would be
wiped out from the vast park within decades. The two arrests
at Deep Creek impressed the reality of this trend on the district
ranger, John Garrison. Garrison had been instrumental in Operation Smokey, a three-year undercover effort to uproot a black
market in bear parts. (Black bears in the Great Smokies were
hunted for their gall bladders, which commanded up to $3,000
each in Asia. Operation Smokey found remains of 368 slaughtered bears and made convictions in three states.) Now Rock
was telling Garrison that the same threat was leveling the park's
rare plants.

When she finished, Garrison and the other officers sat there
stunned. They had been blindsided by another huge and complex market descending on the park.

DEEP CREEK LAY ON the opposite side of the park
from Janet Rock's cabin, on the southwest edge, just outside
Bryson City, North Carolina. A sign beside the road leaving
town said ROAD TO NOWHERE. If you asked someone, they'd tell
you the name is a jab at the government and leave it at that.

In early October Bryson City looked quiet, and life on its
main street was returning to normal after the summer hordes of
tourists had moved on. The barbeque restaurant had only a few
customers, mainly regulars. Outside, on a handbill stapled to a

telephone pole, there was a drawing of ginseng root and the announcement that someone was paying good money for it. The handbill didn't give a name, but it said you could find him on Friday afternoons in Lester's sporting goods shop. I stopped in at Lester's down the street and asked the burly guy with the beard if the 'sang buyer only comes on Fridays. Yep, he said.

"Same guy as last year?"

"Yep."

"How long will he be around?"

"Every week until there isn't any more, probably."

At that point I got a look that informed me I had exceeded an outsider's quota of questions. Locals knew they could find the buyer's pickup some evenings in the supermarket parking lot, or beside the recycling shop on Route 19 out toward Cherokee. You didn't need to ask a lot of questions, and the buyer wouldn't ask you where you got your roots.

The rangers at Deep Creek did ask questions. Their job protecting the park and its visitors involved handling the occasional camper's snakebite, but also investigating crimes on park land. A snapshot on the Deep Creek station's bulletin board showed a ranger standing next to a marijuana plant the size of a tall Christmas tree. *I'll take that one,* the caption said. Not long ago marijuana growing was a major money-making venture in remote parts of the park. In parks across the country, gangs staked out large crops of marijuana visible only on aerial photographs.

"Used to get a lot of marijuana in this park," said Lamon Brown, "but aerial surveillance whacked the big gardens pretty heavy" in the early 1990s. "We were just killing 'em. Now it's either small patches or indoors." These days, ginseng poachers far outnumber the marijuana growers.

Lamon (rhymes with Raymond) wore a Smokey-the-Bear ranger hat on his shaved head and a moustache that bushed around his mouth. Still, he looked too boyish to sound so hardened about criminals. His face was smooth and untroubled as he explained how marijuana growers used GPS receivers to find their patches of weed, or how local gangs had switched from outdoor marijuana patches to stovetop meth labs in their kitchens, which were more cost-effective for "cranking out more product." Lamon said it was common for outlaws to take to the park for refuge, just as it was common for a sheriff's department to get a report of someone fleeing a vehicle or leaving the scene of a domestic dispute. Sometimes people bolted into park land. However, the high-profile manhunt for suspected serial bomber Eric Rudolph focused on the town of Andrews, thirty miles west. The FBI never searched the park for Rudolph; they felt certain he would stay near Andrews. Years later a rookie local cop found him behind a grocery store in Murphy, about an hour from Bryson City.

Lamon grew up twenty-five miles south of Deep Creek. When he was a boy, his grandfather led him to a grove of walnut trees behind his house and showed him a patch of ginseng that the old man had transplanted from the woods. Lamon understood that this was risky. If word got out that his grandfather was growing ginseng, people would slip in and dig it up. After that, Lamon developed a ginsenger's eye.

He told me this late in the afternoon as we walked up an old Indian trail from the Deep Creek station, deep into the woods.

Lamon carried a daypack containing his tools for an all-night stakeout: camouflage jacket, rain jacket, some food, a seismic intrusion device, night-vision goggles, citation book. A layer of dry leaves underfoot made a sound like radio static. A swale on his right started low and rose to a high ridge.

"They love to hunt and ginseng-dig this area," Lamon said. Often he would come here prepared for a solo stakeout, but this evening I was coming along, too.

Lamon knew how poachers think. In the last days before the ginseng leaves disappear completely, diggers scramble to gather up a pound here and there, for that two- or three-hundred-dollar Christmas bonus. Their favorite time is dusky-dark, when there's still enough light for them to see the plants but not enough for them to be noticed by others. Serious poachers will backpack deep into the park, dig for days, and hike back out with fifteen or twenty pounds of ginseng in their pack. To avoid meeting a ranger on the trail, they'll lay low until three or four a.m., then hike to a trailhead, where they will rendezvous with their driver at a prearranged spot. It's planned as thoroughly as a bank job getaway: synchronize, pull up, get in the car and go. Lamon had enough of the criminal in him to understand that poachers simply enjoy the game. He sympathized with their preference for spending a day in the woods digging ginseng over a day on the job. "I mean, it's a beautiful time of year to be out in the woods," he said. "If they can make a hundred dollars in a weekend, it's just a bonus."

Some distance above where he planned to settle in, Lamon stopped and pulled out a canister that looked like a small propane bottle tied to a tent stake. It was a seismic device that worked like an early warning system. Stuck into the ground near a foot trail, the stake was a sensor that picked up vibrations as small as footsteps; the canister converted these to audio signals, then transmitted them on a direct communications channel to the receiver on Lamon's belt. It gave him a three- or four-minute heads-up if anyone was coming down the trail. Lamon hid the stake under a fallen branch and brushed leaves over the tether. A mechanical voice said, "Bleeight." Lamon told me to walk up the trail fifty yards and walk back. The monotone voice said: "Eight, eight, eight."

He adjusted the device's sensitivity setting, then we walked back down the hill and left the trail to find a place where we would sit for a good part of the night. To some, devoting this ranger's time to catching plant poachers is an extravagant waste of taxpayers' money. There are more violent crimes than digging roots in the forest, after all. Park officials respond that in nine years, ginseng poachers stole some $5.3 million worth of root from this park, and the long-term damage is profound.

Lamon saw it from the victim's point of view. "The ginseng and the bears don't write complaint letters."

We waded slowly through the brush in the late afternoon light, and I scanned the ground in vain for root. It was the first week of October, and most ginseng was already down. The chances of my spotting 'sang on my own this season were diminishing fast. I saw black cohosh, but when I approached what I thought was ginseng it turned out to be Virginia creeper.

As we sat at a spot overlooking the path, Lamon said, "There's that ginseng, right there." He kept his gaze locked as he got up, and came back holding a yellowed two-prong stalk. He had found it just by its empty bracts and a single yellow leaf.

We settled into our patch of woods and waited.

The previous week, rangers at Deep Creek arrested a poacher out on Lakeview Drive about this time of day. Two officers slowed down near a car parked almost in the road. As they approached it, a man scrambled up the embankment clutching a big four-prong. He had just dug eighteen plants in full daylight. One ranger said she was glad there were still some dumb ones out there.

Usually it's a lot harder. Every time, the rangers have to build a case from the ground up. Before making contact with a person, they have to establish a reasonable basis for suspecting that person of being a poacher and must be able to articulate those reasons. Trawling the park's roads, glancing at embankments, they watch for torn-up patches of soil or a vehicle that appears to be lurking. A woman driving a pickup back and forth on a park road may be looking to pick up her poacher husband.

For ginseng, probable cause usually means a person with dirt ground into the trouser knees, dirt under the fingernails, and a stick ground off at one end. If someone comes down a path in camouflage pants, with pockets bulging, acting nervous, that's probable cause. An officer will ask a few questions, pursuing any inconsistent answers with more questions. If the inconsistencies multiply, the person may be asked to empty their pockets or open their knapsack for inspection. If they say no, the officer might seize the knapsack and apply for a search warrant. At that point, the officer must be able to articulate very good probable cause. If the judge denies the request, the officer must give the sack back to the person and call it quits. But if Lamon makes an arrest, there are other decisions. First, he must decide whether to bring the accused into the station or issue a citation for them to appear in court later. If they're not a flight risk—that is, if they're local and they have a job—then they receive a citation and are released on their own recognizance.

AN ARREST LAUNCHES AN involved chain of events. The arresting officer must process the evidence, which can mean driving the seized roots forty-five miles across the park to Janet Rock and briefing prosecutors at the U.S. Attorney's office in Bryson City. "Basically, you're educating the U.S. Attorney's office on how much damage this actually is," Lamon explained. "Some of those folks, they're prosecuting rape and murder, and they see a few roots, you know?" The officer has to spell out the long-term effects of poaching, that it can cause a plant's extinction and a hole in the ecosystem. The prosecutors sift the evidence for points to make in court. Sometimes they ask for photos to be blown up; these will be placed on a tripod in the courtroom, along with a map of the region. During the trial, Lamon would point to the map to indicate such things as point of contact, location where the root was found, escape path, and point of arrest.

It had gotten almost silent. We listened to a vague rustle of sounds above the stream's purling. Lamon took a pinch of tobacco and occasionally let a discreet squirt fly to his left. In the distance came what might be a radio, or voices in a higher register. Maybe I was just spooking myself. I asked Lamon if he heard something.

"You, too?" he whispered. "I thought the water was playing tricks on me." His ears were clogged from a cold, so he kept turning to me to see if I reacted. He asked if I could say for sure that I had heard voices.

"It sounded a lot like voices," I said, and imagined repeating that on the witness stand. It sounded equivocal, uncertain. What I heard was like the distant hum of talk radio several rooms away.

The noise seemed to move up the facing ridge, as if someone was traversing the slope. Lamon thought they would either work their way across to our left and come down the path, where they would set off the seismic device, or they would come down to a narrow wooden bridge below us. Up the draw to our left, I heard a low hum. It may have been men's voices.

The day's last sunlight scaled further up the trunks of tulip poplar and maple. Two young oaks stood near us, dark, thin vertical slashes. In the quiet I watched one leaf fall from the topmost branch, all the way down, down, down, until it hit the forest floor. Fifteen seconds. Not long. But only here, with hours to kill, would I watch it all the way.

I kept listening. In the absence of other stimuli, the sounds created almost a delirium.

"This is prime time," Lamon whispered.

A decade ago rangers couldn't get a ginseng conviction even when they caught a person red-handed. Either suspects would fling the evidence deep into the woods, or they would reach the park boundary before they got caught, making it hard to prove that the root came from inside the park. So the rangers in the Great Smokies honed their detective skills more than most park rangers ever need. They learned how to track poachers' footsteps back to the ginseng patches, and how to make casts of bootprints. In ideal conditions after a rain, they could follow the prints right back to a patch of ginseng. In one case, they did that and found ginseng tops lying beside a hole, so they photographed the tops and analyzed the photos down to the color of the soil, noting how exposed soil dries out and turns lighter in color. They made casts of the bootprints. No old-time plaster of paris: they used fine-grain, high-quality dental pumice that fills every nick of a boot's tread.

Lamon leaned forward for a closer look at my boot. An irrational worry flickered across my mind: Was I a suspect? "Look, like this right here," he said. "See where that chunk of rubber is gone? Right here?" Lamon called the leaf-shaped nick in my Vibram sole a "positive identifier."

Covering the vast area of the Great Smokies, the park rangers also used informants when they could. A jealous digger would occasionally rat out a rival, but more often the informant was close to the poacher. "Believe it or not, sometimes your best informants are the guys' wives or girlfriends," Lamon said quietly. Maybe the men neglect their families. Maybe the women want their husbands caught, "so they would quit that foolishness and spend a little more time at home."

One day the park got an anonymous tip from a caller who said that three men—she named them—would be crossing Fontana Dam with ginseng on a certain day at four p.m. The rangers at Deep Creek were skeptical, but Lamon drove with another officer to the dam and set up a stakeout. By four fifteen, three men walked across the dam. All three had loads of ginseng in their backpacks, totaling fourteen pounds.

• • •

As darkness settled, the tree trunks fused into a lumpy gray mass. Lamon unzipped his sack and pulled out a pair of custom-looking binoculars. Some years after the park started night patrols, rangers received military night-vision goggles. Lamon now held a pair with aperture settings that let him adjust light sensitivity and focus. He also had an infrared unit like a slim penlight that could boost visibility on starless nights. The glow of a cigarette a hundred yards away burned as bright as a flashlight. With that, officers could identify someone at twenty-five yards even on an ink-black night. Lamon could track poachers by their flashlights, holding off from using his own flashlight until he got close enough to give chase.

"You want to be close. You want to be close," Lamon repeated slowly. "Try to get your hands on the guy with the gun."

For Lamon, no case was more vivid than four days he spent on the north shore of Fontana Lake, at the park's western edge. It started from another anonymous call. "Somebody had given us a dime," he said. "A couple of fellas were in there digging ginseng." The caller gave a time frame when the two men would be coming out to the lake shore.

"What we *don't* know is *how* they're going to get out—if they're going to come out on a ferry with the ferry service, or a boat pickup. So we spend about three days just staking out that trailhead in there. It finally comes around to the pickup morning and we haven't laid eyes on these guys.

"We figure we had picked the wrong place. So we've gotten up a little before daylight and staked out the trail again going down to the lake, where they've got to get picked up. An hour after daylight we're thinking, 'Well, we've missed it.' So we start panicking."

They creep down to the lake shore. Lamon's partner crosses into the next wooded hollow. "And there they are on the bank, in behind a log, kind of hiding. Waiting for the boat to come in and pick up. And there's a pillowcase behind a tree," he said, pointing to a tree near us. "About that distance, too—about twenty feet above them. And here's a clear path in the leaves up to that tree, and there's a pillowcase, and the pillowcase is full of ginseng. They spent a week in there digging ginseng.

"We immediately separate them. My partner's got one guy over there, and I'm over here talking to this guy, you know: "You don't have to talk to me, but your buddy's over there. He's talking to this guy, and we're going to compare notes. And whoever gives us the truth, we'll pass that on to the U.S. Attorney's office. It would be good to cooperate.'

"So this guy looks at me and he says, "Well, you got us, don't you?'" So Lamon's man sits down and writes up what happened. "Right there on the spot, just spilled the beans." He jots down details of when they came in, where they dug, and where they camped each night. Meanwhile Lamon's partner hasn't gotten anything from the second man, the brother-in-law of Lamon's man. When the brother-in-law learns of the confession, there are words exchanged and threats of beatings. With the confession in hand, the rangers give both men mandatory citations to appear in court and let them go.

The defendants got a jury trial. The written confession made prosecutors confident enough to charge the two with Lacey Act violations, a serious charge that allows for a jail-term sentence.

Although the government lawyers didn't plan to press for prison time, the Lacey Act charge entitled defendants to a jury trial and they got one. The confession was entered as evidence.

Lamon continued: "But then these two guys take the stand and my guy takes the stand and says, 'Yeah, I told him all those things but,' he said, 'I was just scared and I told the officer what he wanted to hear.' And the other guy got up, put one hand on the Bible, raised his other hand, and says, 'I don't know where that ginseng comes from.' Said, 'It wasn't ours.' Said, 'I don't even know what ginseng looks like.' Sat there and told a big pack of lies. And the jury bought it, and found them not guilty.

"You spend maybe four days out there in the woods, eating peanut butter," Lamon said. "You make a good case and then you spend all the pretrial time—a lot of time and effort—and then you lose it. It's part of the game."

Fontana Lake remains a favorite locale for serious ginseng poachers. Typically they will get a friend to ferry them across with their gear, drop them off, and come back for them four or five days later. The poachers set up a base camp and hike deep into the north shore forest. These multiday expeditions can haul out many pounds of root.

The lake sits on top of a deep sense of betrayal, older than the park itself, going back to the 1930s when the federal government came to these mountains with big plans. To create the park, the government used eminent domain and negotiated with each family to buy their land. For some families, no doubt, it came as a boon in the Depression's darkest days. Their land was too steep for crops, their shacks shook with every cold wind, and they suffered from tuberculosis and other diseases. "A lot of these people were tired of trying to hack out a living out of a rocky piece of land," Lamon said. People in the most remote hollows were probably surprised and glad to receive the money and leave.

As part of the arrangement, the government offered to move family cemeteries across the lake onto more accessible land outside the park, or leave them in place and give families access to them by ferry or a road. The displaced families elected to leave the cemeteries where they were and have a road built along the north shore. A dam was built and the lake reservoir filled, with the understanding that the north shore road would be built.

Years passed but no road appeared. Eventually the government built six miles of road out of Bryson City. At that point, however, they struck an unusual acidic rock formation while tunneling through one slope. The rock, when cut, leached acid into nearby streams, killing salamanders, fish, and other wildlife. Tests proved that the Park Service had walked into a quagmire. Finishing the north shore road would cause a wildlife disaster in a national park, but not finishing it would cause a rift with the park's neighbors. The road project stalled.

Children of the families who sold land to the government had regrets. They saw that what had been a steep rhododendron thicket could now be sold to retirees as mountain real estate with pristine views. In Lamon's words, "The government took great-granddaddy's land, gave him twenty dollars an acre for it, and that's just highway robbery."

Today the landscape of old farmstead ruins and the lingering debate give the lakeshore a haunting presence. "You can almost see some old-timer sitting on his porch in his overalls and smoke coming out of the chimney," Lamon said one night as we drove along the park's edge.

A few minutes later he stopped the truck. The headlights shone on a big hand-lettered sign facing the road: ROAD TO NOWHERE, A BROKEN PROMISE, 1943–?

This history colors local views on the ginseng rules, too. In a survey of diggers in the next county west of Bryson City, most felt the government was biased against diggers (many of whom are poor) and inconsistent in how it issued ginseng licenses. A typical comment suspected the Forest Service of misusing license funds and not reinvesting in ginseng restoration. Others complained about haphazard changes in the rules. The report concluded that "past government actions resulting in the displacement of local families from their land" reinforced people's worries about ginseng and other issues "fundamental to their livelihoods, traditions and rights."

Ray Hicks, a nationally famous storyteller in these hills, gave poetry to that tradition. "I lived my life here studying God's creation," he said in his eightieth year, and affirmed that ginseng hunting was as much a part of that study as storytelling. "I just hit a lick when the time of year come for each one: keeping a garden, working engines, gathering the herbs in the forest and telling stories."

AS FAR AS DEFENSE attorney Russ McLean was concerned, Lamon's Fontana Lake stakeout reflected the government's arrogance. He recalled one ginseng case where the Park Service was so sure they had a conviction that they alerted TV stations to have cameras outside the courthouse, ready to report the guilty verdict. McLean stood on the other side, arguing for the defendants, who were Cherokee. McLean told me he had handled more ginseng cases than any other lawyer in western North Carolina or Kentucky.

We talked in his Waynesville law office, where a four-foot-high statue of Justice stood with her foot pressing down on the head of a large snake. Hunting prints and certificates lined the red wall behind his black leather chair.

"They never did catch the Indians, they never saw them," McLean said of the Cherokee case. Instead, the rangers found bootprints in ginseng patches, made castings of those prints, and confiscated the boots of the three suspects. "Tried to claim that these were the boots that made the tracks they had found at the ginseng patches. The problem was, half the people in Haywood County and Swain County and Grant County all wear pretty similar boots."

A former game warden on the Cherokee reservation and two codefendants were charged in that case with four counts of violating game conservation and national park regulations. They were released on bail in February 1994, and in late May the jury trial began in the Bryson City federal courthouse. The jury deliberated about an hour before finding the three not guilty. Park officials were publicly embarrassed.

Behind all that government effort, McLean suspected a desire to prevent anybody from making money off of park property. He also believed the feds held a grudge against the Cherokee for siding with the Confederacy. That's right, he said: the Cherokee fought for the South and as a result lost a thousand acres of their land after the Civil War ended, more than any other tribe. "They're the only people, besides Robert E. Lee," he told me, "who actually ever lost any land because they sided with the Confederacy."

After his three clients were acquitted, McLean said the government started using "this dye thing."

ONE DAY AMID THOSE cases, John Garrison remained in the back row of the courtroom after another set of poachers had been acquitted. A frustrated Garrison turned to Jim Corbin, a biologist with the North Carolina Department of Agriculture, and said, "What we need is a way to demonstrate to the court definitively that these plants came from the park."

Corbin took up the challenge. With a background in biology and as a sheriff's deputy on narcotics cases (his friends called him "half mad scientist"), Corbin plunged into his garage laboratory. (Corbin also once ran a Christmas-tree farm, and was, briefly, a running back for the Washington Redskins.) He came out with a method for marking the roots of ginseng plants within the park boundary. He modeled his plan on a practice from wildlife management on the West Coast, where biologists used wire inserts to mark clams. When seized by law officers, the marked roots would be solid physical evidence that the ginsenger had dug inside the park.

Corbin experimented with different types of markers. He tried tiny metal i.d. chips on which he punched a near-microscopic code in Navajo, a language he knew from several years as a missionary in New Mexico. When injected into ginseng roots, the chips were invisible until X-rayed. This worked fine technically but was useless; Park Police rarely had X-ray facilities. So Corbin tried combinations of bright orange dye, injections of calcium and magnesium, and metal and silicon filings. When mixed in a powder with minerals calcium and magnesium, the dye was absorbed quickly into roots as if it were food.

The dye proved a success. Dyed roots not only gave the rangers physical evidence against poachers in court, but the bright orange dye that suffused the roots took even unapprehended poachers out of the ginseng trade. As Corbin liked to say, "Nobody's going to buy a ginseng root that looks like a Tennessee football jersey."

Corbin has dyed roots in nearly every ginseng patch within the park's boundaries, an effort almost comparable to planting Manchuria's Willow Palisade. The process involves finding the plants, carefully unearthing them, sprinkling the dye on the roots, and replanting them. Some time ago, Corbin estimated that his team had logged fourteen hundred miles on the ground, marking roots. Not surprisingly, he knows Bob Beyfuss. As we hiked through woods near the park's Smokemont campsite looking for root, Corbin mentioned that he met Beyfuss years ago when they were both working on ginseng physiology. "Bob's really enthusiastic," Corbin drawled. Had I seen Beyfuss' ginseng tattoo? The tattoo no doubt showed well because Beyfuss kept in shape and "liked to wear skimpy-looking stuff."

Corbin spent a summer in the Deep Creek district working alongside Lamon Brown: each day, they hiked fifteen to eighteen miles through all terrains, unearthing roots, dyeing them, and moving on. The task quickly amplified the competitive element inherent in ginsenging. The two men found themselves racing to find the next 'sang patch.

"It's a competitive area, when you stick a little testosterone into the equation," Corbin said. "You get the fever hunting it."

When asked about Corbin, Lamon just smiled and said, "Jim's kind of a humorous guy after you've been around him a little bit."

With Corbin's dyed roots, night-vision goggles, and the dental pumice for footprints, the rangers' arsenal for evidence was growing, and the battle between the park and the poachers was escalating.

"In Southern Appalachia it's always been so much more intense." Corbin saw his neighbors' obsession with ginseng as a kind of addiction. "That seems to be the one weakness of these folks, is that they just *can't stand* somebody else getting it," he said. "It's who gets the biggest plant."

"And why is that such a temptation?" Corbin asked. "Why go to the federal penitentiary for digging four pounds of ginseng?"

"Try to get your hands on the guy with the gun," Lamon told me. By now it was full dark. I wouldn't be able to see a gun in front of my face, but Lamon said the night-vision binocs would help.

"If you're stationary and three or four guys are coming in through here with some hunting dogs, you get a visual on which guy's got the gun. You know you ain't going to get all four . . . so you want the guy with the gun. Then you've got a good, solid hunting charge."

If you're lucky, you lay hands on someone's collar as soon as the words "police officer" are out of your mouth. Lamon demonstrated that grip in the air.

"If a foot chase ensues, if he gets out of sight around one curve," he warned, "the gun's *gone*." Two syllables for emphasis. "He's going to pitch it, or he's going to keep on burning shoe leather for the boundary."

The same strategy applies to ginseng poachers: If three guys make like a covey of grouse and scatter in all directions, lay hands on the guy holding the bag of 'sang. He will be the fastest one. The decoys walk in front to draw out the law. If a badge appears, the runner takes off. "If he can get hid, he'll shove it under a log, put some leaves over it, and he'll mark it by that double tree right there." Lamon pointed out an accomplice tree. "He'll walk on out, let you contact him. 'Why'd you run for?' 'Ah, man, you just scared me.'"

IN JANUARY 1996, a Bryson City man named Harold Laws was tried for ginseng poaching, and Russ McLean was in his corner. Laws was caught red-handed, carrying roots dyed orange. The jury deliberated less than forty-five minutes before declaring Laws guilty. He received a sentence of six months of real prison time and twenty-four months probation. That conviction and several others caused a downturn in ginseng poaching, said the park rangers.

In some cases, the government seeks restitution for the cost incurred in replacing the seized roots, including the drive that Lamon Brown must make to take the roots to Janet Rock's plant morgue at Twin Creeks. There, as she has done many times,

Rock takes the evidence to the basement, weighs each root on an electronic scale, and counts the neck scars to estimate its age. Most are five to nine years old; occasionally she sees a thirty-year-old root. The oldest was forty-eight years old. If they're still viable, she puts them in the fridge for replanting later. If they're too far gone, she'll dry the roots so that rangers can use them for educational presentations, or for undercover operations to catch dealers buying out of season. Then there's always the possibility that the suspect will be acquitted, in which case the roots are returned. So far, that's never happened.

Janet Rock monitors a rich tapestry of rare plants throughout the park, from log moss to black cohosh. She loves them all, but she concedes that her favorite is ginseng. It's always hovering near the brink of extinction. "There's a lot of mystique to it," she says. "It's exciting when you're out looking for it and you find it, and you have a hunch you're going to find it. You see plants that it likes to grow with, so you slow down."

She, too, has helped Corbin with the tedious work of marking the roots against poaching, and she agrees that ginseng itself injects adrenaline into the work. "It's always a thrill whenever I take technicians with me, when they start to learn to identify it," she says. She watches for all its forms: from seedlings with only three leaflets, to the summer's flush of red berries, the distinctive pale yellow in the fall, a bare-stemmed four-prong. Like Lamon, she keeps tabs on the buying price.

Replanting the seized roots back where they came from can mean returning them to the same hollow, possibly the exact spot where they were untimely ripped from the earth. Occasionally a poacher will tell where he collected the root and rangers will put it right back in that spot. So the convicted poacher might do time in a cell and then go on with his life, while the stolen roots might spend months on ice, and then return to theirs.

WHEN IT BECAME CLEAR that we had been hearing only phantoms, and that we weren't going to catch any poachers that night, Lamon and I walked back to the truck. We drove along the park border beside Fontana Lake to check another spot. It was a moonless night and the darkness was complete. He pulled to a stop on the road's shoulder, where I could just make out, in the truck's headlights, a bridge beyond a bank of rhododendron.

"This is it. This is the road to nowhere," Lamon said. He cut the engine. "If it were daylight you could see the beginning of the tunnel past that gate." The tunnel with no exit. This was where two poachers had been apprehended. Lamon described the flight of one of them into the woods, the arrest, and a night-long vigil to protect the scene until incriminating evidence— two bags of roots, marked by bright orange dye—could be retrieved at daylight. It had meant another sleepless night for Lamon. "Some people just enjoy the game," he said.

NINE

Tamed, but Not

*What a story roots of this age could tell of the passing
seasons—of storms, drought, forest fires, and escaping the
roving eyes of the ginseng hunter. Most remarkable.*
—Val Hardacre, *Woodland Nuggets of Gold,* 1967

The Marathon County airport in central Wisconsin lay in
the middle of a farmland platted with gray silos and
ponds, quilted at the seams with woods that by October had
turned yellow and orange. Black-and-white dots were spattered
across the still-vivid green dairy pastures. Long, straight two-
lane roads stretched into the distance, empty. There were few
clues that this was a national bull's-eye for ginseng growing. But
it was true: America's ginseng industry was centered in Wausau,
and locals said the airport was built for the ginseng industry.
Marathon City, a quiet town nearby of under two thousand residents, was home to two of America's leading ginseng exporters
and many of its largest commercial ginseng farms.

The county's preeminence was due to a quirk of history and
a few individuals. In the last decades of the 1800s, with the

Industrial Age in full bloom, scientists decided they could re-fashion ginseng from a relic of wilderness and irregular harvests into an engine of trade and economic vigor. Progressive agricul-turists set about taking the root out of the forest and sending it forth in orderly rows, like other field crops. In the 1880s J.W. Zahl was among the first to tinker with growing ginseng, on his farm in Antigo, an hour east of Wausau. Around that time, in upstate New York, a retired tinsmith named George Stanton was doing the same thing, building wooden shade arbors and laying out regular rows that could be weeded and sprayed with the efficiency of a modern farm. Stanton planted six thousand ginseng roots and another ten thousand seeds and hoped his ef-forts would pay off. The plants survived, and his neighbors caught on. Stanton organized his fellow New York ginseng farmers into an association, a move that sparked imitators else-where. He wrote articles that fanned interest in growing ginseng nationwide, and became known as the "father of cultivated gin-seng." Seeing the growing demand, the U.S. Department of Agriculture published an 1895 bulletin on how to raise the plant, then a full manual eight years later. As the twentieth century dawned, ginseng gardens, as the farms were called, were sprout-ing up across the land.

GINSENG RISING IN VIRGINIA! trumpeted the Richmond *Dispatch*. The old view that ginseng could never be cultivated, the paper reported, "has been exploded," and growers were get-ting three dollars a pound (equivalent to about sixty-two dollars a pound in 2004) for their new crop.

Perhaps it's remarkable that it didn't happen earlier. Ginseng is an angiosperm, the group of flowering plants that have come to dominate the world's flora and have been generally amenable to domestication throughout history. Angiosperms bear their seeds in a protective ovary, and so for most of them, reproduction is relatively easy to influence. Yet ginseng stayed wild, and its demanding site requirements pushed would-be shang farmers to extraordinary lengths—they put seeds in aquarium sand and kept it moist for a year just to get them to germinate; they built shade structures and planted seedlings in beds raised off the ground to ensure the drainage and airflow the finicky roots demanded. Population biologists categorize species according to their life-history strategy. R-strategist species act like weeds: they're fast-growing and often short-lived to take over new habitats quickly. (The *R* stands for reproduction as a priority.) K-strategists, on the other hand, tend to be slow-growing and long-lived, and focus their energy on maintaining a place in their native habitats. (The *K* refers to carrying capacity and the fact that their habitats are more stable.) Ginseng is a K-strategist that requires, as one botanist puts it, "very exacting agronomic conditions for cultivation."

In April 1901 a teenager in rural northeastern Ohio named Val Hardacre watched out the schoolhouse window as a neighbor hammered away on a bizarre structure in his backyard. Later the boy asked his father about it and was told it was shade for a new crop. "It's called shang around here," his father said, "but the correct name is ginseng."

The next morning Val stopped on his way to school and asked the neighbor for a look at the thing. No plants had pushed up through the dirt yet, but the mysterious shade arbor haunted him for weeks. Val knew he wanted to grow shang, too.

Before long he was trawling the woods, looking for the plant that was worth a dollar a pound, a fortune for a boy at that time. He and a friend finally found a small plant in the forest; the root was just a few inches long, but they were ecstatic. "Lady Luck had smiled on us that June day," Val recalled years later. More ginseng hunts followed. He would race home and show his finds to his father, who would look the plants over, occasionally expressing surprise at where his son had found them. "Boy, you have a dollar's worth there," he'd say. "Dr. Cowles is buying all the plants he can get."

Soon Val was paging through *Special Crops* and *Ginseng Journal,* magazines devoted to the ginseng enthusiast. The ginseng business was booming and old-timers were already afraid that it was "poised on the brink of ruin and over-exploitation." George Stanton wrote that "boomers and sharks" shouldn't overwhelm the business; he cautioned growers not to share their ginseng seed.

Nonetheless, the boom got a little crazy. Thieves burgled ginseng gardens. Some went to prison. Insurance companies started issuing policies that covered ginseng crop theft. *Special Crops* published an account of a 'sang thief in Virginia who was electrocuted by a fence installed by a grower. The body was left to rot for a week before it was buried. "[H]e sleeps on there in peace," the grower wrote, "and my sleep is more peaceful, too, for I'm not afraid of my ginseng garden being robbed any more."

For Hardacre, what started as a treasure hunt gradually became something more. In the vocabulary of his taciturn family, ginseng expressed a bond that he would soon miss. His father died when Val was still in high school, a crushing blow to the large family. The son realized that his father's energy and quiet passion for the outdoors had come through in their talks about ginseng.

He soon tended a ginseng garden of his own (along with a factory day job) and spent weekends tramping the woods searching for wild plants. Hardacre was not a naturalist or a man of letters, but an ordinary citizen with a strong sense of wonder. He became proof that although farmers had taken ginseng's mystery out of the forest, they still believed in that mystery. Eventually, when his own mortality loomed closer, it was the story of ginseng that Val was moved to tell more than his own. In his eighties he published *Woodland Nuggets of Gold,* a book that weaved world history and his life story together through ginseng. It rises almost to poetry when Hardacre reflects on the oldest plant he ever dug, a sixty-year-old wild ginseng root. "What a story roots of this age could tell of the passing seasons," he wrote. "Most remarkable."

Instead of demystifying ginseng, the business of cultivation added another facet of fascination. It was like grafting the appeal of the stock market onto an already seductive activity. Novelty ventures sprang up to manufacture ginseng chewing gum, ginseng ice cream and ginseng toothpaste. In 1926 the New York firm of Wm. J. Boehner & Co. set a new gold standard of farmers' hopes when it bought a crop of ginseng from the Fromm Brothers of Marathon County, for $107,388.75. For the Fromms, the sale represented a yield of over $16,521 per acre. It was the largest single purchase of a ginseng crop ever.

Then came the Great Depression and global unrest. When

the Japanese quarantined Chinese ports in the 1930s, the ginseng trade came to a halt and the number of American ginseng farmers dwindled. Even after World War II ended and commerce resumed, doomsayers warned growers that they were being exploited. Often American growers received less than a seventh of the price their roots fetched in Hong Kong. A government botanist cautioned that ginseng was not a gold mine, and farmers shouldn't expect a great return for their labor and capital. Hard-core growers didn't listen to him.

WISCONSIN REMAINS THE largest source of cultivated ginseng in the United States, and nearly all the state's ginseng farms are in Marathon County. People in that part of the state still tend to think big about the ginseng business and aren't scared off by a bumpy ride. A few months before my visit, a former Marathon ginseng farmer had launched a soda for mainstream markets. Bottles of *Ginseng Rush* were lined up on Wausau grocery shelves, and the company was preparing to expand nationwide. Then bad reviews brought a swift end to the enterprise, for the time being.

If the small-time ginsengers in Appalachia had their idiosyncrasies, I soon found that the industrial-scale folks had their own. The day after I arrived in Wisconsin, I was summarily dismissed from the grounds of the country's second largest ginseng exporter. Their facility was several miles outside Wausau, past large silos and old farm houses and newer suburban homes, on a narrow road among the fields. Through the doorway of a large white warehouse I could see the telltale brown barrels. The office echoed emptily as I entered, and a woman told me the owner was very busy, but she walked with me toward the ware-house and called to a heavily built man in overalls, who had his back to us.

He turned and there was no mistaking his bearish posture or his menacing silence. He wore thick glasses and appeared to be in his fifties, a farmer of northern European stock like the Fromms. I was writing about ginseng, I said. Could I get some information?

"What? No." Then: "Forget it. *For-get it!*"

He stomped off toward the warehouse. As I drove away, the Neighborhood Watch signs around the property warned IF I DON'T REPORT YOU, MY NEIGHBOR WILL!

I SPENT SEVERAL DAYS in Wausau, and one morning met ginseng farmer Randy Brunn in a coffee shop when he was running late. His truck had frozen the night before and wouldn't start. He asked for ginseng tea but the waitress said they didn't have any. (He orders it in every café he visits, but only one in ten has it.) He settled for Earl Grey.

Brunn got bitten by the ginseng bug twice over: when he was a boy, his grandfather used to take him into the forest to dig for wild roots; and then as a grown-up he stumbled onto Marathon County's farming secret.

He had grown up two hours west of Marathon County but he had never heard of ginseng gardens and their riches. In 1975, after finishing college, he moved to the county for a new job. Driving through the farmland that summer, he noticed strange structures in the fields. Under a lattice roof eight or nine feet high, sometimes under plastic, gardens looked like a hybrid of a greenhouse and enclosed farm. The full-leaved plants, nestled together in long, unbroken rows of green, hardly resembled their thin, wild relatives in the forest.

"When I came through town the first thing I wanted to know was, 'What's all these pheasant ranches?'" he said. They're not pheasant ranches, people told him; they're ginseng gardens.

"It was a pretty closed lot, like mink growers or cranberry growers. They kind of kept to themselves. And even in those days you didn't hear a lot of Wisconsin ginseng talk. It just wasn't in the papers," he said. It wasn't in the libraries either. *Bright with Silver,* a book by Katherine Pinkerton about the Fromm Brothers and their farm, still gets stolen from the county library, and used copies sell for up to $150 each. Randy recommended I read it if I could ever find a copy. (Back in Connecticut I did find a copy in the deep reserve of my local library, but it could only be read under the watch of a librarian.) The four Fromm Brothers began as furriers in mink and fox in the town of Hamburg. International buyers for their furs came from Russia and the Far East and stayed in Wausau's Landmark Building. It was a small step to attract international ginseng buyers, too, so around 1915 the brothers added ginseng gardens to their land. The Fromms were patient, methodical men. They tinkered with shade methods and designed elevated beds for good drainage and better airflow. They mulched their shang beds in winter months, and treated the seed in a way that improved germination. They hired housewives and teenagers for the labor crews needed to work their hundred acres, and built dormitories for some of the workers.

The Fromms remained patient through the Depression and

China's trade quarantine. They stored their ginseng during the war years (raising silver foxes kept them going through the 1940s) and waited out world events.

"They had just a mountain of ginseng root in one big granary on the floor," Randy said. His eyes went distant. "I lost my train of thought," he said.

Like the Fromms, Randy's family came to Wisconsin from Germany in the late 1800s. His grandfather Hugo Singerhouse grew up in a large family and dug root. When Randy was about six years old, he came across a bunch of muddy, wrinkly roots upstairs in his grandparents' farmhouse, spread out on newspapers that covered the floor.

"Here he had all these roots laid out, and I asked, 'What is that?'" Randy recalled. "'Well, that's wild *ginsheng.*'" The dirty things looked like carrots or turnips or parsnips. Back then, his grandfather dug several pounds of root every fall and got forty to fifty dollars a pound. He also dug wild goldenseal. The old man taught him what to look for in the woods, how to dig the root, how to put seed back in the soil.

Randy forgot all that until he discovered the shang gardens of Marathon County. Then he decided he'd grow some ginseng himself, but it took him three years to find out how to do it. He couldn't find anyone who would talk about it or sell him any ginseng seed, so he asked his grandfather to show him again how to find it in the woods.

"I said, 'You'll have to take me in the woods and show me what ginseng looks like.'"

He followed the old man through the forest as he casually pointed out ginseng and goldenseal. Back in Marathon Randy prepared his garden. He hammered together shade structures for a couple of acres, plowed the land five and six times before putting in the roots. There were other tricks you had to know, including the history of your farm, because you could never plant shang on the same soil twice. It was such an intense plant that a single crop exhausted the soil's micronutrients for growing ginseng. There was also what Randy described as "a disease complex," caused when ginseng infects the soil with its own particular nemesis. Nobody knew exactly what caused this, but the result was that if you planted a second ginseng crop even fifteen or twenty years after the first one on that site, it might grow well for two years but by the third year it would wither from root rot. With root rot, you don't see the damage until it's too late. All your roots turn to mush in a week under healthy-looking leaves and stems. This situation turned Marathon County's cropland into a minefield.

"No one knows the magical answer to it," Randy said.

The waitress brought his tea. "It's too bad the industry has gone where it's gone," he said, steeping his tea bag.

Back then, Marathon County felt like the center of the world. Big firms like Boehner & Co. would buy large orders based on a single sample. Buyers flew in from New York and China, including two men whom Randy called Uncle Ho and his nephew Chung Ho. Those two by themselves would buy up nearly half the crop. Paul Hsu was getting big then, too.

In early October the buzz would start: "Uncle Ho is coming to town."

"We'd get a little nervous," Randy said, "because he was the most revered one. Everyone would bow to Uncle Ho." Uncle

Ho installed himself at a table in a local café or cafeteria, where growers would bring him their roots and he would decide how much to pay per pound. Sometimes growers managed to get buyers into bidding wars, taking advantage of the fact that the buyers tried to wrap up purchases by the weekend so they could send the shang air freight the following Monday. Flying Tigers offered three-day air freight service to China.

Wet weather ruined the crops during a disastrous three-year stretch in the mid-1980s. The next fall Randy and his wife decided not to harvest their ginseng, to keep their three-year-old roots in the ground for another year unless the price got above thirty-five dollars a pound. In mid-October, the demand suddenly surged over that threshold. They harvested very late, almost the end of October. The roots came out of the ground nice and big: chunky, clean, three-year-old roots.

At this point in the story, Randy seemed to vacillate between a fascination with the biology and the adrenaline of the deal recollected.

"We had three buyers bidding on it," he said. "We started at thirty-eight dollars." The bids went to forty, forty-one, and continued over the weekend. For two nights he and his wife lay awake, wondering, "Do we take it or don't we?" At forty-one dollars a pound the bidding stalled and finally one of the buyers offered forty-one and a quarter. The Brunns sold to him.

The next year the price jumped again, to over sixty-two dollars a pound. If you had a ton of roots per acre, you got a return of over a hundred thousand dollars for that acre. Randy had three and a half acres. Those were salad days. Randy and his wife and family all worked together. Farming was fun. "You could afford your insurance, your labor, take a trip to Vegas if you wanted to."

Sure, there was risk. One year a grower in western Wisconsin had an excellent crop of eleven-year-old roots that he was finally ready to dig. He had invested ten years of labor and sweat in those roots, with a beautiful crop of ginseng to show for it. "I'm sure he's got pictures," Randy said. Then root rot came and wiped out ninety percent of the crop. If that farmer had harvested a year earlier he would have made a small fortune. Randy couldn't stop thinking about the pictures. "Just imagine an acre, just a forest full of big, green plants with big red seed heads on it. Beautiful!"

Then the word got out that Wisconsin's ginseng farmers were making over a hundred thousand dollars an acre. That was the threshold that put it in the newspapers. A few growers started selling their ginseng seeds to outsiders, and there was the convention. I remembered David Law: "That damn convention in Canada! That was the biggest mistake they ever made." When Law had mentioned it, the event sounded like a miscalculation, but Wisconsin farmers spoke of the convention like a blind right hook that had left them reeling. David Law had an aerial view of the disaster; Randy Brunn experienced it like a close-up shot.

In the mid-1990s the problems mounted along with the price of fertilizers and fungicides needed for battling diseases like root rot and rusty root. Soon it cost $35,000 per acre to grow ginseng on farms, yet the market price for farm-grown roots continued to decline. Then came competition from Canada on a big scale, and year after year of too much rain. Farmers could no longer cover their insurance premiums. One grower described the downturn this way: Back when he started growing ginseng in the late 1960s, you could buy a new Mustang for $2,000, and he made sixteen times that much off an acre of ginseng. Now an acre of ginseng farm didn't yield enough to buy one *used* car.

Banks stopped lending to ginseng growers. Buyers stopped coming around. Farmers switched to other crops or bought dairy cows. Banks foreclosed on a number of farms and growers had to take jobs in town. At that point, Randy said, there was bitterness.

Randy scaled back his own ginseng operation. His daughters had no interest in farming ginseng now, and he and his wife were phasing out the last acre. But Randy hadn't given up. He was getting into simulated-wild ginseng, planting it in deep pockets of forest where people wouldn't look.

THE BIGGEST GINSENG GARDEN operation in Wisconsin, and one of the largest in the country, belonged to Paul Hsu. Mid-morning in the warehouse of Hsu's Ginseng, just north of Wausau, found him dressed in a dark blue suit, crisp white shirt, and red tie, kicking the top off a ginseng barrel for a Korean television crew. The top didn't budge.

"Not enough karate," he joked. He took a step back and prepared to launch himself at it again.

Paul Hsu has achieved success by attacking problems and taking chances. My first impression of him was cued by the high-end cell phone, wire clipped to his shirtfront, and the new gold Mercedes. His unlined face made him a young-looking sixty. Against a background of midwestern farmers and insurance businessmen, Paul Hsu stood out.

Hsu grew up in the Pescadores, a hardscrabble archipelago in the strait between mainland China and Taiwan, islands where people grow peanuts and sweet potatoes in dry, stony, treeless soil. His parents were farmers who thought Paul, the seventh son, was destined for the ministry. His grandfather had been the first in his village to convert to Christianity when an English missionary came through.

"I'm sort of the favorite," Hsu said, then corrected himself: "I *am* the favorite." It's the only time he sounded less than self-assured, almost embarrassed.

As a young man he did not hear the call of the church. He worked with a U.S. Air Force project that brought medical supplies to the Pescadores, and found he enjoyed it. He decided to study social work, which in hindsight he sees was a compromise between the ministry and business. He met a young woman named Sharon at church, and asked her to go with him to Denver, where he'd been accepted in the University of Denver's social work program. He applied for a scholarship from the state of Wisconsin, which was granted with the condition that after he finished his master's degree he would spend two years as a social worker in Wisconsin. That was how a young man from Taiwan found himself in a state clinic in Fond du Lac, Wisconsin, counseling Midwesterners on domestic troubles and how to get out of debt.

Fond du Lac was where he heard about American ginseng. Few people in Taiwan knew anything about American ginseng; it was just an herb that came from Hong Kong. Hsu had early memories of ginseng's tannic scent, and he recalled his mother taking ginseng tea after each of her children was born, to help restore her strength. By the time she reached her sixties, after fourteen children, her mobility and digestion were poor. Friends suggested Paul send some ginseng home to her, so he sent home a handful of Wisconsin roots. When he visited his parents six months later, he saw that his mother's color had improved and she was moving around better than before. They said it was the ginseng. Hsu returned to Wisconsin resolved to find out more about shang farming.

He said, "I started because it helped my mother," a story tailor-made for marketing. But learning about the business was even harder for him than it was for Randy Brunn.

"Everybody took the Fifth Amendment," Hsu said of his efforts in the early 1970s. Everywhere he went in Marathon County he ran into stone walls, and he still had obligations in Fond du Lac, three hours away. But after a visit to the Fromm Brothers' operation in Hamburg he started to think that maybe he could make it in the ginseng business. He could become a direct link between American farmers and the Taiwan market, bypassing Hong Kong. His first order came from his younger brother, to send thirty pounds of root to Taipei.

That started Paul Hsu's career moonlighting in ginseng. He learned the business at night while handling domestic disputes during the day. Soon he was considering leaving social work and jumping into the ginseng business full-time. His parents thought the idea of ginseng as a full-time job was ridiculous. "You've got a good job with the government," his father said. "Why would you want to give that up?"

Sharon, now his wife, supported them with her nursing job while he got the business started. It was 1974, they had a newborn, and Nixon was hanging on to the presidency. In the fall Hsu worked seven days a week, often from seven a.m. until ten at night, buying root from farmers at the receiving dock of his warehouse and at their fields. He set up pickups and deliveries and established a system for taking purchase orders, shipping orders, organizing grading and packaging, making contacts with exporters, and marketing. He claims to have been the first Chinese-American business to get a toll-free phone number and run a mail-order operation in the United States.

He did everything himself for two years, then he hired a secretary. His brother ordered more shipments and helped out by sending payment up front. Growers helped by giving him thirty days from date of purchase to revolve funds. A Wausau bank gave Hsu a small-business loan. The 1970s weren't good for most small farmers, but it was a good decade for ginseng growers. So in 1978 Hsu decided to become a grower as well. He bought farmland north of Wausau, although he was only four years along as a dealer, and his family's farm background in the Pescadores didn't help. He had no experience with farm machinery.

Other growers felt threatened by Hsu's shift from dealer to grower. They thought he was trying to cut them out of the market. Hsu farmed over a thousand acres of ginseng, the largest cultivated ginseng operation in the country. As the market heated up, he felt more competition at the other end, too. Hong Kong buyers who had bought from Hsu soon began buying straight from farmers, cutting *him* out of the chain. A few who spoke English best became his direct competitors. In 1987 Hsu's last major Chinese customer, with whom he had dealt for ten years, stopped buying from him.

That's when Hsu decided that if they were coming to Wisconsin to compete with him, he would take the competition to Hong Kong. The social worker turned to hardball. It wasn't enough to be a major exporter and a big farmer in America's Dairyland. He began strategizing about how he could break into Hong Kong's tight-knit circle of Cantonese ginseng importers, whose families had controlled the business for generations. Hong Kong had enjoyed a lock on ginseng imports to Asia at least since 1949, when Mao Zedong closed the mainland ports to foreign trade. After that, American ginseng went into Hong Kong and was smuggled into Guangzhou or up the South China coast. A fraction of it got shipped elsewhere in Asia.

The Hong Kong players had generations of experience and contacts that kept the industry concentrated in a few hands. Hsu's main competition was (and remains) a handful of large companies in Hong Kong, including Sun Ming Hong, David Law's company. Hong Kong's wholesale ginseng importers are centered on one street—Wing Lok Street—and they all belong to the ginseng graders' guild, a subset of the Ginseng and Deer Antler Association. For decades, these importer-exporters held silent auctions among themselves, bidding on the containers of American ginseng that entered the harbor. They smuggled most to the mainland but the rest went to Singapore, Malaysia, and elsewhere in Asia and Australia.

Hsu had no entrée into Hong Kong. He didn't even speak the language (having grown up speaking Mandarin, not Cantonese). But he banged his head against the door of the graders' guild for four years, trying to get into Hong Kong because he knew it was the opportunity of his lifetime. And beyond Hong Kong lay the vast mainland.

Finally, in the early 1990s Hsu opened a branch office in Hong Kong, and in December 1993 he negotiated to ship twenty thousand pounds of raw ginseng roots straight to the mainland port of Ningbo. China was opening up and Hsu was getting in. The next year he shipped a third of all American ginseng that went to Asia. The company's sales topped $18 million.

Not everyone was happy with Hsu's mainland contacts. His father's generation was wary of China. Still, many educated Taiwanese of Paul's generation saw that reunification with the mainland was probably inevitable. Hsu expected that in a few years over half of Taiwanese businesses would have investments in China.

In the warehouse outside Wausau, the Korean TV crew was shooting Hsu's employees at work. In an airy room, seven Hmong women in red aprons sat at three tables, each using clippers to trim roots for different categories. The atmosphere was one of quiet industry, and the only sounds were the snap of the graders' clippers and the low music of their conversation. In the wide window behind them, sunlight poured over a cornfield. The occasional red leaf of a weed in the field echoed the workers' red aprons. Korean interest in this scene is understandable, since ginseng has been important there for nearly as long as in China. Korea was a hub of trade in *Panax ginseng* with China and Japan at least since the 1700s, and Korean farmers have cultivated Asian ginseng on a large scale (along with other medicinal plants) for over a century. At last count, twenty-two thousand households in South Korea were growing ginseng on

over fifty thousand acres of land. Wild ginseng, practically extinct there, is a curiosity for TV viewers.

Then Paul Hsu was standing in a smaller room full of
drums. "This room is all wild," he said. The cameraman
aimed his Sony Digital 1000 down on six open barrels of wild
roots. Hsu explained that he exported five thousand to seven
thousand pounds of wild ginseng annually. He looked into
the lens and said, "Wild ginseng is going to get more expensive every year."

PAUL HSU SEES HIS place in history. He may be the
first big ginseng dealer to integrate his business from farm to
wholesale export, to retail mail-order sales, to Hong Kong and
China imports, and further to have retail kiosks in cities like
Shanghai. Because he saw his opportunity as historic, he continued with Nurhaci-scale persistence to scramble over formidable
hurdles, entering first the Marathon County clique, then the
Hong Kong circle. (He put his Hong Kong office just a few
blocks from the ginseng graders' guild.) He spent over a decade
getting into mainland China, and says it was worth it. He is one
of just five or six major players in the China market and the last
one to enter before it hardened into its present division of market share.

THERE WAS ANOTHER, lesser-known factor in Marathon County's ginseng boom in the 1970s and 1980s. True, the
Fromm Brothers had established the methods and knowledge
among farmers in that part of Wisconsin, and yes, demand
from China had risen. But a third factor was Wausau's Hmong

community. With the end of the Vietnam War, central Wisconsin saw an influx in Hmong refugees, an ethnic group native to the mountains of Laos. During the war thousands of Hmong had helped the CIA cut off North Vietnamese supply lines. When the American army left Vietnam, Hmong hopes for a free homeland faded, and most were forced to flee. The Hmong in Wisconsin provided a pivotal labor force for a crop as labor-intensive as ginseng. Few people credited them, Paul Hsu said, but without the Hmong it's unlikely that the state's ginseng farmers could have sustained their production at a time when people were leaving farms. Ginseng gardens require an enormous amount of hand labor: weeding, picking seeds, sorting roots, and of course digging. You can't pull a combine through a shang garden. "For this, people have to get down on their hands and knees," one farmer told me. "It's a wet, cold, miserable bloody mess." Most Americans wouldn't take such work, he said, but a generation of Hmong immigrants had. How had they gathered here, in central Wisconsin? Did they know ginseng in their previous lives in Asia?

The Wausau Hmong Association occupied a small, white professional building in a neighborhood just east of downtown. Abraham Yi Vang, the executive director, is also small and professional. He stands under five feet tall, but his shoulders fill his size 42 tweed jacket, set off by a green lapel button. His moustache is trim and his wave of black hair makes his square face look much younger than his fifty-six years. But what strikes you when you meet him are the petite but strong brown hands. Almost delicate.

On one wall of his conference room hung the largest story

quilt I have ever seen, roughly eleven by thirteen feet. Hmong story quilts (often just two feet square) use a traditional Hmong form to tell a story of modern displacement. They depict in embroidery chilling scenes from the Hmongs' exile from Laos: airplanes drop bombs, camouflage-wearing soldiers fire machine guns into huts, and tiny figures desperately swim a wide river to crowded refugee camps. There was something of that epic formality in Vang's quiet voice when he began to explain how Hmong came to be involved in farming American ginseng.

"So when we arrived in this new land, most people were very interested in becoming farmers," he said, "because in Laos they had self-sufficiency to support their own family." But why Marathon County?

He started again: "I came from a refugee camp to the United States in 1976 and lived in Memphis, Tennessee, for seven years," he said.

Vang grew up in the hills of northern Laos, about fifty miles from the Vietnamese border. The terrain was high and the climate was cold enough that morning could bring a frost that lasted until the sun was high. There were very few level places for growing field crops like rice. Most Hmong families grew food for their own subsistence. They used all types of plants. Some looked like potatoes, he said, but they were red, blue, many colors. For medicine, too, Hmong used local plants— roots, herbs, and shoots they found in the forest. But Vang never saw ginseng in Laos.

One of his grandmothers, an expert herbalist, could treat eye problems, wounds, and even chronic heart disease with plants she found locally. If a person's illness required a root, she'd go into the jungle and find it. Abraham saw her heal knife wounds with an unguent. When she fled Laos she took with her plants for medicine. Vang was nine or ten when his grandmother treated a man who had been confined to a wheelchair, a teacher from the lowlands. Their village had no schoolteacher, so a Hmong elder ("one of my grandpas," he said) rode his horse down to the nearest lowland village, outside Xieng Khouang, to bring back a teacher for their children.

"So my grandfather let this Laotian teacher ride the horse, brought him to our village. He came to our village for four years and my grandmother looked for the natural herbs to treat him. After four years, he went back to his hometown. He was walking strongly then." The rehabilitated teacher became a school principal back in the lowlands, but every year, in gratitude, he came back to their mountain village to visit Vang's grandmother.

From 1967 to 1969, Vang worked with the U.S. military along the Vietnamese border, leading a team of twenty-four Hmong, who monitored the movements of North Vietnamese troops and supplies southward on the Ho Chi Minh Trail. He maintained round-the-clock radio contact with bomber planes, guiding them to their targets based on his group's reconnaissance. The planes lit up the night.

Vang later moved to an artillery regiment near the border and was reassigned to Long Chang, the CIA's base of operations. For his collaboration with the Americans, he and over a hundred thousand other Hmong were forced to flee across the Mekong to Thailand. He was processed through refugee camps and ended up, along with other Southeast Asian refugees, in Memphis. There he found work installing carpets, delivering appliances, and other odd jobs. He saved enough money for vocational courses and got a job at a factory that manufactured water pumps.

Vang had been in Memphis seven years when one day his aunt and uncle suddenly appeared at his door with a U-Haul truck. They said they were taking him to Wisconsin. They, too, had come through the refugee camps, but ended up in a larger Hmong community in Wausau. "Better you move to the north," they told him. "Stay with us."

So they loaded up his belongings, and he moved north of Milwaukee. In Wausau, Vang saw opportunities for Hmong self-sufficiency. Gradually he found his place as a community leader. He was astonished that the climate felt like home, or at least more so than Memphis. "Here the weather is cool," he said. "The weather is not so different from Laos."

He even thought the hills outside town might hold plants like the ones back home. Such things had happened before. If the plants were there, he knew his grandmother the herbalist would recognize them. She had spent days at a time in the Laotian jungle and knew all the many-colored fruits and tubers.

"We tried to take her to the forest so she could see which ones were the same as in Asia," he said.

You can imagine them, their car parked on the shoulder near a stretch of woods. Two younger men follow their grandmother hesitantly as she looks up at the maples, birches, butternut, and black ash. She scans the grasses and vines on the ground, hunting for one that knits this place to their first home. Maybe she tilts her head and squints, the way Dave Cooke regarded Jilin's forests, with the men following her the way that Randy Brunn trailed his grandfather into the woods looking for ginseng.

"She said no, totally different," Vang said. "She couldn't find any kind."

With no familiar herbs nearby, the Hmong in Wausau adapted to ginseng and other local alternatives like goldenseal and echinacea. Sometimes they found what they needed in Asian grocery stores in Chicago's Chinatown. Vang ground ginseng roots into a powder for tea, or for soup, and he boiled it with chicken or pork and served it with rice or potatoes. "After six months, your body feels healthy," he said, pumping his arms. "When you walk it's almost like you're hopping." In the winter he'd drink a cup of ginseng tea and then go out and shovel snow without feeling cold. He'd also put a fresh root in a jar of drink; it lasts longer and you can have it anytime you want.

WAUSAU HAS THE HIGHEST concentration of Asians in Wisconsin, and most of them are Hmong. There are Hmong radio stations, bilingual newspapers, and restaurants. *Future-Hmong* magazine has articles on how drivers can avoid hitting deer and how car insurance works. Until recently fifteen new Hmong families moved to the area every year. (*Wausau* is the Sioux word for "faraway place," which seems particularly apt for a Hmong sanctuary in America.) As executive director of the Wausau Hmong Association, Vang spent a lot of time persuading authorities not to punish Hmong for practicing their traditions. Animal sacrifice, for example, could pose problems. But Vang alerted doctors and police officers to Hmong culture and tried to calm the waters when, say, a shaman slaughtered a pig.

You had to make special arrangements. In a hospital, you had to talk with doctors to get permission for a shaman to conduct certain rites. The Hmong association also filled needs left unmet by the U.S. government, which has never repaid them for their wartime service. Most Hmong want to become farmers, Vang said, but they don't qualify for bank loans or government assistance. Vang's challenge was working with local agencies to help families become self-sufficient. "Self-sufficient" was his mantra. Hmong were used to living independently in remote mountains, so life in a society as interconnected as America was a massive adjustment. To be branded as freeloaders added insult to injury. So Vang arranged job training and English-language courses. The association offers computer classes downstairs and Hmong language classes upstairs. There were workshops for preventing domestic violence, for helping young people avoid gangs, and for learning about Hmong culture.

Farming in Wisconsin was different from Laos, but he knew what was needed to grow ginseng: land, machinery, certificates for applying fertilizers and pesticides. Market contacts. Those were the hardest. You could grow vegetables and take them to the local supermarket and they would say no. They wouldn't buy yours because they have a contract with other producers. That made many Hmong lose hope.

"They said, 'Well how are we going to survive in this land and support our families?' We don't want to rely on public assistance because our cultural history is not that way . . . So we said, 'Well, it sounds like in Marathon County ginseng is what is popular in the market.'"

Vang estimated there were sixty to seventy Hmong families growing ginseng in Marathon County, with more coming from elsewhere as seasonal workers. Many came from the Twin Cities and spent the summer. The numbers were declining, but Hmong still farmed over a hundred acres of shang, and they would go up again if the price rebounded. Vang himself was farming three to five acres about ten miles away from his home. He recruited his family—children, nieces, nephews—and traded his own labor with his friends. His children didn't like going to the farm. "They hate it," he laughed. "But there are times, you can say, 'Well kid, I need your help because I need more labor. Help me.'" His oldest son was twenty-nine years old and worked in a Wausau factory.

Vang's ginseng harvests had been down for three years. Too much rain and cold. Rain, flood, root rot, and rusty root. From nearly two thousand pounds per acre in a good year, harvests had dropped to under a third of that. Buyers might visit his garden and say that his roots were too long, or not "chunky" enough.

"I see people quitting ginseng growing," he said, "but I don't see any other crop that they can grow to replace it." He knew that potato farmers made marketing deals with Burger King and McDonald's, but how could Hmong growers compete with them? He also tried growing ginseng in the woods, but that takes even longer to pay off.

AMONG THE SHANG FARMERS that I met in Wisconsin, only one appeared unconcerned with the power of the buyers. Lyn Heise said he married into ginseng. He learned about the business from his wife, Germaine, who was growing a small patch when they met in the early 1960s, when Marathon County had only about forty growers.

The Heise farm stood on a red-dirt road twenty minutes outside Wausau, a few acres snugged up against a forest. As I drove up the driveway, I passed the ginseng patch: a nondescript acre of land covered in plastic, studded with wooden slats. Seasonal workers had just finished that autumn's harvest. Heise came out and met me at the door.

"Probably ninety percent of the work is still hand labor," he said. "At harvesting you want maybe thirty workers. You want to get it done in one day." Heise acknowledged he has relied a lot on Hmong labor.

Like all ginseng farmers, the Heises used extreme measures to fight root rot, sometimes sterilizing the soil to kill disease, sacrificing all the plants in the process. One year seemed disastrous: the seed was slow to germinate, the plants were buffeted by unseasonal winds and then by hard rains. The plants looked terrible aboveground, but when it came time to harvest, they got a bumper crop—about three thousand pounds an acre. "Everything went wrong, and it was the best crop," he said. "I didn't think there would be anything, and there were huge roots, as big around as a half dollar." Heise liked the unpredictability.

Inside he showed me the other reason he and his wife stayed in the business. About twenty years before, they discovered they could gain leverage against middlemen by processing ginseng into capsules and selling it themselves. "Now we're not at their mercy," he said. "If anything, we're their competitors."

"We bought a few health magazines and we saw this was the big thing," he said. "No matter which one you bought, it always had the capsules."

When they went into ginseng manufacturing, other growers thought they were crazy. The huge investment in processing equipment and marketing, with no ready distribution contacts, was unheard of. But the Heises found that manufacturing opened possibilities for getting a much better price for their ginseng and bypassing the wholesale bottlenecks. They filled the first batch by hand, grinding the roots into a powder and filling one capsule at a time. It took them a day to make five hundred capsules.

Later they got a machine that could make thirty thousand capsules an hour.

The couple placed only one ad, in a small magazine in Texas. Ever since, customers have found them through distributors or by word of mouth. They now have a large mail-order clientele and have figured out how to use even the pencil-thin roots that are the least profitable part of the market. The Heises sell them as Ginseng Chews. "People love them! Nobody else in the world has them, except us."

Heise led me through the barn-size processing room, with its shiny metal sorters and packaging machines. The customized equipment was expensive. He always had to keep several months' worth of inventory on hand to fill orders, so he had barrels of roots in the entrance, raw material ready to be ground into capsules.

As we came out, he paused before the small sales display case. Amid the chews and boxes of capsules, Heise pulled out the most valuable item there: a gnarled root shaped like a person: arms, legs, everything. He had been offered five thousand dollars for that root.

Lyn Heise couldn't say exactly what had gotten him into ginseng. Certainly curiosity was part of it, but as a former accountant he was more pragmatic than most ginsengers. He had gotten as much control over the plant as he could, from forest to farm to manufacturing and sales. But he still respected ginseng's surprises. Describing the plant's dormancy, he said, "If they think the year's going to be crummy, they won't grow." He caught himself. "I know they don't think—*people* think." Still, it was easy to forget.

American ginseng couldn't quite stay put in America. Whether it was an Appalachian hillside or a Midwestern farm, someone was always prodding it to leave the soil and move on.

TEN

Shanghaied Once More

Members of the public are reminded not to bring endangered species into Hong Kong without a license . . . Statistics showed that items commonly seized from travellers at customs checkpoints include orchids, cacti, American Ginseng roots, crocodile meat and crocodile leather products.

—PRESS RELEASE, Agriculture, Fisheries and Conservation Department, Hong Kong, 2002

December was halfway over, but David Law had not yet shut down the engine for the season. He was shipping out about eight hundred pounds of root every Friday from JFK. Wild roots had been coming into his office from Kentucky, West Virginia, the Blue Ridge, North Carolina, Ohio, and Wisconsin. (The company's office in Canada handled most of the cultivated harvest.) On the phone he laughed and told me he was buying a little more than he probably should, but he felt he had to ride it. Law let me tag along one Friday as he took another shipment to the airport.

All through the fall, people had told me surprising things. One Wisconsin grower mentioned, in passing, that the ginseng trade sometimes involved a black market in slaves between Hong Kong and the mainland. "Ginseng goes in and slave labor comes out, usually girls," he said. "So it's ginseng in, girls out." This guy had been a ginseng grower for decades; presumably he knew a few things. He added that smuggling American ginseng along China's southern coast was common, even legitimate. China was the only country he knew, he said, where smuggling was a profession. "It's as legal as being a writer," he said with an open hand toward me, "nothing wrong with it."

I considered that as I once again made the walk from the Astor Place subway station to David Law's place in lower Manhattan. The streets were flush with commuters—a man in a suit with his tie loosened, ready to be tightened for a nine-o'clock meeting, a nurse in whites lighting a cigarette against the cold on the way home from his shift. The rapid click of heels. The morning sky was pale gray, almost translucent. The neighborhood's shops were opening: Curry in a Hurry, Spice Corner, a nail salon, an Indian bookstore.

Law came to the door looking transformed from when I had seen him in September. Instead of an urban boho, he now looked like a woodsman dressed for a hunt: jeans, flannel shirt, a quilted hunting vest and a dark wool hat with narrow brim and earflaps over a new short haircut. He invited me inside for a cup of coffee before we left. A Christmas tree stood in the living room, not yet decorated. A carved wooden display case held several vases, a graduation photo, and Mariah Carey's latest CD.

Law's youngest son, James, rumbled down the stairs in pajamas, blinking.

"Where's Kenny?" his father asked.

"In his room. Should I wake him?"

Law said no, they could handle it. He went out and pulled a two-tone blue Astro minivan around front and set its flashers going as the morning rush filed down Lexington Avenue. He and James soon had the drums on the sidewalk and were loading them through the cargo door. The van's backseats had been removed, and a sheet of plywood reinforced the floor. Law raised each barrel with a practiced leg move that seemed to save his back, then James rolled each one back into position. Law prodded him to tighten up the arrangement. Soon all eight drums were in.

This happened every week. "It's become a ritual," James deadpanned as he swept sidewalk trash into a dustbin. He was still wearing his pajamas under a windbreaker. "This," he said, nodding toward the trash, "is a fifty-dollar fine."

Law smiled. He put a black briefcase in the cargo well and we pulled away from the curb. We slid down Third Avenue and eddied onto Broome and then Mott. We stopped first at a Chinatown bakery that Law ran with one of his brothers. When he came back to the van he handed me a piece of sponge cake in wax paper.

Crossing the Williamsburg Bridge toward Brooklyn, slices of the East River passed between the girders below us. Law told me about the fights he had with his own father back when he started in the ginseng business. His father had started working in a Hong Kong ginseng shop at sixteen, eventually opening his own store that sold ginseng. David made the mistake of selling one of his first shipments to his father.

"Oh boy. I got screamed at," he said. "Man, I got so much

negative reaction, right? I felt so *ashamed*! I should just quit the damn business." This made him erupt in laughter. "You know how fathers can be. The most difficult person to make happy is your father."

Many years later, his father admitted that the shipment had actually been very good.

"'Now you say that!' I said, 'Look at me—during that time, you knew how vulnerable I was, right? I just started the business, right? You were my second customer!'" Law laughed again. "That was terrible."

We passed into Brooklyn. A few minutes later he assured me that his father was a nice man, just strict; he demanded the best from his children, more than they could accomplish. Law thought a bit. Maybe he was too demanding of his children, too, he said through a bite of sponge cake.

Back when Law was still working at the airport and trading in ginseng on the side, everything—cultivated and wild—went to Hong Kong by air. But since the price for cultivated had dropped, it now went by surface, either shipped through the Panama Canal or by train to the West Coast and then by freighter to Hong Kong. If you time it right, a surface shipment gives you two months of storage free, which becomes significant when warehouse space in Hong Kong's harbor gets expensive.

The wild stuff still went air freight. He'd take the load first to customs for inspection of his CITES paperwork. Each drum of wild ginseng had to have a certificate from the state of origin. Law jerked his thumb over his shoulder and said that this batch contained roots from Virginia, West Virginia, Carolina, and Kentucky. He had some from a buyer I had talked with in

North Carolina, and two drums from Tom Cook's bunker at Anglers Roost.

I craned around again at the drums riding behind us. The lid of one said, in magic marker, 'TCWV.' Tom Cook, West Virginia. For a moment it seemed that some of these roots were chasing *me*.

"Nice guy," Law said. He has dealt with Cook for many years. And yes, Law had talked this season with F.G. Hamilton, the nonagenarian dealer in rural Virginia. Hamilton, with his hermit ways, was still an important buyer, and honest, Law said. Too bad that ginsengers sometimes took advantage of the old man's blindness.

There was one question I had asked everyone that season, about the price of ginseng. Was someone really driving it up? Rangers in the Great Smokies insisted it was high, one of them suspected a cartel. Everybody from Janet Rock to Bob Beyfuss had heard something, but nobody knew for sure. Dave Cooke in West Virginia didn't know what hiked the price. Jeanine Davis was tracking trends among Carolina dealers and saw some curious patterns, but she wouldn't hazard a guess.

Did David Law know who had driven up the price?

He looked straight ahead down the lanes. "I believe it was probably me," he said. "I was the bad guy." He backpedaled a moment, mumbled something about other factors. But after another minute's pause he came clean.

Law had begun the season with several thousand pounds of last year's root in his basement. If the price went up, he knew, that inventory could make an extra fifty dollars a pound. So maybe he offered a little more per pound for this season's harvest; that price would also float his inventory. Ordinarily Law handles between 10 and 20 percent of the total market; this year by being aggressive, he probably dealt with a quarter of it.

"That's how we play the game," he said. "Sometimes your inventory hurts you because the market goes against you. Sometimes your inventory helps you, if the market goes with you." He had jumped in and pushed the market higher, but other big dealers helped, too. He didn't think he could do it alone. "You've got to weigh the situation," he said. "Sometimes it works out."

We were approaching Hangar Road. "Just do it," he said, a little giddy from the confession. "You know what Nike says? Just do it."

He pointed over to where inky smoke was rising from near a runway. They were testing the fuel, just as he used to when he worked for Allied Chemical. "That's JP Four," he said. "For prop planes. See? They put it out." The smoke billowed black, then disappeared.

Just then we reached the big, green perishables building. U.S. CUSTOMS SERVICE, it said in silver letters above a bank of windows. Two men in inspectors' uniforms stood at a mobile snack truck buying cups of coffee. The large parking lot stretched away from several lanes that led to loading docks, and all the lanes were occupied.

"Oh shit," said Law. "We've got to wait."

At least since the early Qing dynasty, bureaucracy has played its role in ginseng's annual migration. In those days the imperial Ministry of Finance regulated the grading process: Roots were sorted by size and shape; those that resembled a human shape were most valuable. Age and place of origin were also factors; older, wild roots with well-defined rings and a fine grain were highly prized. Ginseng gathered later in the fall was judged more valuable than roots dug earlier. All roots were to reach Beijing by the twelfth month of the lunar calendar, in time for the New Year celebration. The shipments were scrutinized by officials from the Grand Council of State, the Imperial Household, chief eunuchs from the Inner Palace, and other supervisors before being shuttled to the palace warehouses.

During the 1700s Qing officials funneled American ginseng from Canton to Beijing through similar channels, although sailors and blackmarketeers skirted the restrictions of the Canton merchants' guild, or Co Hong, with furtive visits to merchants' shops.

Later came the U.S. Food and Drug Administration, the Fish and Wildlife Service, the state departments of agriculture or forests, and the Foreign Agricultural Service, which tracks exports of cultivated and wild ginseng roots (a third category for simulated-wild was recently introduced). U.S. exports for both wild and cultivated ginseng have declined, for different reasons. In addition to the competition from Canada, growers and markets also sprouted in Europe and Latin America. How do you explain a $67,000 spike in exports of farm-grown ginseng to Guadeloupe one year? Or the $31,000 cache of wild root spirited to Mexico in 1999? Neither country showed any interest in the years before or after. There was also a Colombia connection: every few years, somewhere between $40,000 and $90,000 of root passed through that country. U.S. exports of wild ginseng have declined at a more gradual pace as pressure on the natural populations have intensified and reached their limits.

Even as Law's minivan approached the customs dock at JFK, the U.S. Department of Agriculture was tracking the year's exports. By the end of December, wild ginseng exports to Hong Kong would spike 50 percent over the previous year, an aberration in a downward trend. As China lowered its import tariffs as a new member of the World Trade Organization, more American ginseng was going straight to the mainland; those shipments totaled over $6.3 million in wild root that year, a fifteenfold increase over the year before. The trend was to bypass Hong Kong and ship directly to ports near Shanghai and along the coast of Guangdong Province. Meanwhile, cultivated ginseng shipments from the United States dropped by more than a third.

Like a vast electrocardiogram, the USDA figures from year to year were charting wild ginseng's vital signs, a complex of ecological decline, shifting demand, and changing tariff policies. Sorting out which factors jerked the needle down could be nearly impossible, but it seemed certain the wild ginseng population couldn't long sustain losing over sixty thousand pounds of plant material every year.

"The better the medicinal plant, the more it threatens its own existence," insisted James Duke, a retired medicinal plant expert from USDA. His statement echoed a saying attributed to Chuang Tzu: "The tree on the mountain height is its own enemy. The grease that feeds the light devours itself. The cinnamon tree is edible: so it is cut down! The lacquer tree is profitable: they maim it. Everyone knows how useful it is to be useful. No one seems to know how useful it is to be useless."

Ginseng being ginseng, part of the trade fell outside legitimate commerce. In Hong Kong, despite repeated official notices warning travelers not to bring endangered species without a license ("The public should pay more attention when buying wildlife products as souvenirs," chided one official), ginseng smuggling incidents were rising, and topped 145 by mid-year. There was also the aphrodisiac sidelight: the *South China Morning Post* noted that Big Spender Sauna, a seamy massage parlor on the Kowloon side of the harbor, was hawking the benefits of ginseng in its spa water and massage oil, although it was "quite debatable whether ginseng osmosis will help Big Spender's customers keep their stamina up." Investigations into gray areas of the ginseng trade in the United States sometimes turned up awkward connections. A man who marketed Gerovita, a pill sold as "Mother Nature's Male Enhancer" that listed Asian ginseng among its ingredients, was convicted of mail fraud but was later pardoned by Bill Clinton in his last days in office. In the 1970s John Chancellor reported on national television that cult leader Rev. Sun Myung Moon owned businesses making ginseng tea, as well as others that sold titanium and Korean arms; Senator Robert Dole, who would later make commercials for Viagra, called for an investigation.

DAVID LAW FINALLY ROUSED the sleeping driver of the Ultimate Express van that was blocking the customs lane, and backed his own minivan into Bay 5. I followed him up the concrete steps to the loading dock, and he was buzzed in through a door. As we pushed through a butcher's curtain of wide, clear plastic strips, one of the inspectors hailed Law. The man was bearded and wore a crisp white shirt with a Customs Service shoulder patch. Law had explained that the Customs Service inspectors here were actually agents for the Fish and Wildlife Service. The inspector sat at a desk in the drafty warehouse and joked with Law; they had running gags that spanned the two decades he has been coming here. The inspector kept suggesting that he and Law should open a kosher bakery together. They would make lots of money.

Law knew the drill. He stepped onto the dock elevator and pressed a button. The platform lowered with a low motor hum to the minivan, where he would pull a drum for inspection. As the platform went down, the inspector seemed to have second thoughts.

"This is ridiculous," the inspector said. He knew that most of the roots had broken necks anyway—it would be impossible to tell if those plants were three years old or ten.

At that point a second inspector came up, a thinner man with a gray goatee. I had seen him at the coffee cart earlier, worrying with a coworker over his son's college expenses. He spoke in the argot of many warehouse workers, a weary and cynical knowingness.

"It all comes down to an acronym," the second inspector said, "IAB." The ginsengers, the buyers, the whole works, he said: It's All Bullshit. "You think the government knows what's going on, because of this rule?" Nope, he said, IAB. "The people who sell it are bullshit, the people who buy it are bullshit. They think it's going to make their shlong hard."

The first inspector offered a mild rebuttal: The aphrodisiac claim was passé. Nobody believed that anymore. "What ginseng is," he said, "is a mild stimulant."

Law didn't argue with them. Untaping the top of the drum, he simply stated what he had expressed earlier in the van: what people believe in, they buy. He had held up a coffee cup to explain: His bakery sells coffee at fifty cents a cup — good arabica, he insisted, better than Starbucks, but much, much cheaper. The eight-cent cup cost more than the coffee. But people pay more for Starbucks so they can believe that it's superior. When Starbucks customers pay three dollars for a latté, they *believe* it's a better coffee. They feel good holding a Starbucks coffee cup as they walk down the street.

Law pulled off the top of the barrel, and the first inspector looked through the plastic interior bag.

"But it's so expensive," the goateed man objected.

"The more you believe in it, the more you pay," Law said. People don't trust a product if the price is too low, he said.

"IAB," said the second inspector.

The customs warehouse seemed an unlikely place to argue the value of ginseng, but here we were. David Law wasn't saying that ginseng was worth its high price because *he* believed in it, or because Chinese medicine had proven its usefulness. Ginseng was worth its price because the *consumer* believed. Law knew he wouldn't persuade these two with Chinese clinical experience, so he was basically staking an economic position that went back to Thorstein Veblen's ideas of conspicuous consumption. But he might just as easily have drawn on the idea behind the Iroquois Thanksgiving Address — that the high price for wild ginseng was a sort of thank-you transaction that recognized the plant's importance for the person who bought it, except that this transaction wasn't complete because it didn't cause any replacement seeds to be sown in the forest (except for any simulated-wild roots that had snuck their way into Law's drums).

The first inspector handed me the CITES forms to look over. The red stamp in the lower right was still fresh: RELEASED.

As we headed for the door, the first inspector reminded Law of his proposal: they should open a kosher bakery in Brooklyn. Law laughed over his shoulder.

"Usually I'm not this lucky," he said outside. Another inspector, Ralph, wasn't there today. Ralph would insist on inspecting the drum that was hardest to reach, the one flush against the driver's seat. So Law would have to haul out ten other hundred-pound drums to get it.

"Whenever he sees Chinese or black or whatever come in he doesn't like, he'll make you suffer," Law said. Ralph would insist on dumping the whole drum onto the floor—usually the biggest drum, 140 pounds of little roots on the concrete floor. It's impossible to put it all back, so Law would end up with several pounds of fragments that wouldn't fit. Larry would say, *That's your problem.* Sometimes he would dump out two drums on the floor.

For that reason Law brings most shipments himself. If a trucker weren't careful and shipped a drum five pounds light, that could kill the trust of a Hong Kong buyer, and Law's reputation would suffer.

"This is still three hundred thousand dollars," Law reminded me, glancing at the eight drums.

• • •

NOBODY SEES PROMISING NEWS in the plant's long-term trends toward extinction in the wild, and yet few involved in the trade have proposed restrictions on wild-ginseng exports besides the minimum-age rule instituted by the Fish and Wildlife Service. Gary Kauffman, the Forest Service botanist, asked, What would happen if the government banned all harvests of wild ginseng, at least for several years? Judging from experience, that could cause a rush of even more intense harvesting. Diggers would think: *Since there's no legal stake in wild ginseng or its future, I might as well take what I can now. I can dig it secretly and get the bonus of whatever the black market will bear.* For cultivated ginseng, on the other hand, it's reasonable to wonder what will happen when China becomes self-sufficient in that low end of the market. It's possible that the transpacific trade in American ginseng will dry up altogether from a combination of wild ginseng's disappearance and a glut of cultivated roots. (Few Western scientists, including Varro Tyler, the pharmocognosy expert, have found any chemical difference between wild and cultivated ginseng, or any significant differences between younger and older roots.) China is cultivating more and more American ginseng, and some predict it will be self-sufficient in farm-grown American ginseng before long.

From the customs dock, Law drove out Rockaway Boulevard to complete the paperwork with the freight forwarder. The top floor office of the air-freight company looked out on brown grassland, a Brooklyn wilderness. Models of China Airlines cargo planes stood on a shelf, nose up, near a row of clocks all set to ten-thirty. Law shared a laugh in Cantonese—about me,

I suspected—with the man at the near desk. He passed a check for the bill of lading.

Law made sure the airbill stated the cargo only in general terms (he would advise the airline about the specifics once the drums were safely onboard and airborne) and double-checked to confirm that the papers did not indicate an insured amount that would attract attention.

As we pulled up to the airline freight dock to deliver the barrels, Law grumbled about the airline. "The service is lousy," he said. He unloaded the barrels from the minivan without ceremony. Law divided the order in two, and I helped him wrestle the drums onto two pallets. In Hong Kong the shipment would be split between two customers: barrels numbered one through four went to one customer, and five through eight to another. We waited for a forklift operator to come.

The warehouse was as deep as an airplane hangar, with blue metal racks rising four or five levels deep. Offhand, Law figured it was big enough to hold $800 million worth of root wholesale.

A bored security guard wandered over to us. "What's inside?" he asked. "Candy?"

"Yeah, powder," Law said.

"For candy?"

"Right. Sweet candy." Law knew of an incident where over twenty pounds of ginseng was stolen through the bottom of a container, in exactly this airport setting. The shipper had carelessly written HIGH VALUE on the box. Law couldn't afford that kind of mistake.

The forklift operator finished his root beer and swung over to impale the first wooden pallet. He rode away. We watched until he came back for the second pallet.

DRIVING BACK TO MANHATTAN, Law told me about his fishing trip earlier that fall. He and his two sons and a friend left the city one Saturday at four a.m. and drove upstate to a remote spot off the Taconic Parkway, a place where Law has fished many times over the years. Near there he owned a shack and ten acres of land where one day, he expected, he'd build a house and retire. His kids had no interest in the place: no television, no VCR. Not even a generator. For now it was adequate for an occasional fishing trip. But that day in early November the fish weren't biting. His sons were cold and bored.

"We sat beside the river for hours," he said, then they gave up. They decided instead to go into the hills and dig ginseng. Law knew those woods and over the years he had broadcast seed on his land. By the end of the day they had dug fifteen pounds of root.

"I haven't dug ginseng for a long time," Law said. "I was surprised to find so much!" They filled four brown grocery bags with roots.

The Manhattan skyline showed through the bridge girders before us, looking functional and unromantic above three lanes of clogged traffic.

"My kids don't even like ginseng," he said. "They like truffles."

As we ebbed back into the city, he grew philosophical. He was getting old, he said, and he doubted whether any of his kids would go into the ginseng business, or even that it would be there for them. But then he stepped back from pessimism. "Coming to America gave me opportunities," he said, his eyes straight ahead. "Gave me a chance. I made a little bit of money. I'm happy."

ELEVEN

Served by the Finest Chefs

Inhale first that wondrous aroma of ginseng root so
that the very first spoonful of this herbal soup will make
your very senses reel with delight.

—TAN BEE HONG, restaurant critic,
Kuala Lumpur, Malaysia, 2001

In the opening sequence of *Iron Chef,* the Japanese cooking series, the show's theatrics are telegraphed in dramatic silhouettes of three gourmet chefs as they rise on pedestals like culinary gods. These gladiators are the Iron Chef masters who face challengers in each episode. Weapons include a primary ingredient and whatever secret ingredients the combatants can marshal in the fifty-minute period. The duels are covered by a team of journalist types, including a breathless reporter on the floor of Kitchen Stadium and commentators in the studio, and judged by critics in the dining room (these usually include a famous actor whose verdict was often "I like this" or "Really tasty"). All of this is dubbed into American English for another layer of surrealism.

One night as I watched, Kitchen Stadium hosted a duel that

ranged across Western and Eastern cuisines. And knock me down if one of the secret ingredients wasn't the bitter, gnarled root. The challenger, grandson of a famous Shanghai chef, used ginseng in a soup with flat, silvery tuna and bird's nest. The judges savored their bites and gave the dish high marks, giving special mention to the ginseng taste.

Ginseng, it turned out, was not simply bad-tasting medicine. Before, I had thought that George Albright's verdict on the root's bitterness was a consensus: barely tolerable. Could that basic experience of flavor vary so much? Could a root that tasted bad on one continent taste good on another?

The question drew mixed responses. A producer for the Food Network, Maggie Shi, had childhood memories of her mother brewing a pot of "bitter, allegedly medicinal soup" and forcing Maggie to drink it. "The only way to tolerate it," she wrote, "is to gulp the liquid down as quickly as possible." Yet still she posted the recipe on Epicurious.com. Her mother's dish mixed together one American ginseng root, one chicken breast, five slices of dried abalone, and five or six cups of water, and got high ratings from people who tested it. Some suggested adding dried dates or angelica root to cut the bitterness. Others said that good health just tastes bad.

In Asia, restaurants from Singapore to Seoul have built reputations on blending that unpleasant tang of good health with more appealing flavors. Singapore's Imperial Herbal, located in the Metropole—a setting reviewers have called "medicine hall demeanor meets avant-garde"—specializes in tasty tonic dishes. Its soups use shark fin with Asian ginseng or codonopsis (a plant that herbalists sometimes use as a ginseng substitute), and astragalus with braised cod. In Kuala Lumpur, one dish at the Shangri-La hotel's Shang Palace sent a reviewer for the *New Straits Times* into rapture. It was a soup served near the Chinese New Year (the name translated as "The Season of Spring Brings Smiles All Around") and reminded the critic of home cooking over a charcoal fire. For her, the "wondrous aroma of ginseng root" set the senses reeling with delight. Hong Kong restaurants serve winter tonics such as hot pot, sometimes called a casserole, in a half-donut-shaped tureen. These use ginseng along with bird's nest, snake, and deer antler.

Ginseng was probably used as a food before it gained currency as a health tonic. In China, tonic cuisine has a long pedigree. Instead of the four basic food groups of Western nutrition, Chinese cuisine generally aims to balance yin and yang. Yin foods are those that cool—grapefruit, melons, star fruit, bananas, and seaweed—and yang foods have a warming effect, like pepper, dried ginger, soybean oil, cinnamon, and ginseng. In between these extremes lie gradations of mildly yin (apples, mangoes, eggplant, strawberries, wheat, and tomatoes), neutral (beef, milk, peanuts, pumpkin, string beans, abalone, pork, honey, and figs), and mildly yang (asparagus, for example). In that tradition, a mother has a wide range of options for picking a dish for her sick child. If she decides he's cold and wet, she might make a yang soup; if he's hot, a sweet yin dessert of poached pears, lemon balm, and honey might help. Tonic soups range from sweet red bean soup, for warming the body in winter, to green mung bean soup, used for acne and skin rashes. You might make peanut soup for long life, or sweet potato and lotus-seed soup as a laxative.

"The relationship between soup and rice is like that between water and a boat," wrote Qing-era poet Li Yu. "When a boat is stranded on a sandy bank, only water can wash it back to the river; rice goes down better with soup." Soups have a strong tradition in Shanghai cuisine, and many recipes for tonic soups that use ginseng have a link to Shanghai.

In Korean cooking, too, ginseng is used in chicken soups and in other dishes. Barbecued ribs are sometimes marinated for a full day in red ginseng and served with fried rice noodles. (Red ginseng is Asian ginseng processed through a special steam-drying procedure that is found at only one facility in South Korea.)

MOST TRADITIONAL RECIPES CALL for Asian ginseng, but as experience with American ginseng has grown, many chefs have embraced it. Filipino recipes for chicken and pork soup advise you to toss in 'sang, red dates, and ginger. An Indonesian recipe for Stewed Bird's Nest includes American ginseng, and Paul Hsu lists a few recipes on his website: for ginseng whiskey, a fish soup with red dates, turkey stuffing, ginseng-banana muffins, tossed ginseng salad (dubious), and sex muffins. In the Chinatown of Washington, D.C., I found ginseng sold at a breakfast counter on H Street, where grits were on the menu and the clientele was mostly African-American.

For most Western palates, though, the root has a long way to go. Energy shakes and smoothies are a step in that direction, and Jeanine Davis, the agricultural agent in North Carolina, has a recipe for ginseng chocolate cake. A farm in Maryland promotes a "wild-simulated ginseng energy shake" along with a recipe for venison tenderloin that they marinate in soy sauce, sherry, and sugar before stir-frying and sprinkling with ginseng strips.

Despite the commercial failure of Ginseng Rush, many other soft drinks and teas have established themselves on the market, including an uncola counterpart: Ginseng Up! "This golden-colored herbal beverage has a mild spiced flavor and a nice bite," one ad notes, "plus it has the replenishing attributes of ginseng." Besides the original flavor, which tastes like lemony ginger ale, the company has expanded its line to lemon-lime, grape, orange, and apple.

Leonita Machado, a manager with the company in Massachusetts, felt sure that Ginseng Up! could take off like Coca-Cola did a century ago. Machado pointed out that Coke, too, started as a health drink, then succeeded by sheer force of marketing ubiquity and sweetness. "This has both," Machado said. "It's healthy and good tasting."

Originally from Quezon City, in the Philippines, Machado was a microbiologist and lab manager at the Ginseng Up! bottling plant, located on a narrow alley in Worcester, the industrial New England town where the first commercial valentine was mass-produced in 1847. Worcester is far from both Quezon City and ginseng country. It's much closer to Mansfield, a town where, in October 1996, the middle-school principal suspended three students for drinking ginseng tea. (The girls believed that the ginseng "would make you hyper," a school official explained. Their plan to reach an altered state, more than the ginseng itself, triggered the suspensions.)

In over a decade with Ginseng Up!, Machado had watched the drink's market grow steadily and leap the divide from marginal specialty shops to mainline grocery stores. Her lab in the Worcester plant had counters along all walls, lined with beakers and small vials of chemicals, as well as crayon drawings by her daughter and her two-year-old son.

Exactly how much ginseng actually went into Ginseng Up! was hard to say. The company imported its extract from Korea (the owner, also from Korea, insisted that Korean ginseng was the most pure). The extract came into port in New York and got trucked up to Worcester in large plastic containers of viscous dark brown liquid. Machado sampled the extract in her lab to check the quality and oversaw the mixing process next door in huge metal vats, where it was blended with flavorings and water. The water was triple-filtered through charcoal, sand, and paper, and then carbonated. The mixture got swirled and piped downstairs and poured into a seamless row of bottles that glide past on a conveyor. The bottles proceeded to a pasteurizing area, where they got labels plastered onto them. At the back of the bottling room, pallets loaded with white cases of the drink were stacked and shrink-wrapped, waiting for the eighteen-wheelers that scraped their sides to squeeze into the company's loading dock and take them to supermarkets across the country and beyond.

NOVELTY DRINKS OFFER A starting point for Western palates, but adventurous chefs have taken the blend of East and West further. In December I talked with Ming Tsai, bestselling chef and Emmy Award–winner for his first cooking show *East Meets West,* and host of *Simply Ming* on PBS. Tsai (pronounced *sigh*) and his wife own Blue Ginger, a stylish restaurant in an upscale Boston suburb that showcases his blend of Eastern and Western cuisines. He has been profiled in *People* and *The New Yorker* as a leader of a new breed. Tsai wears his celebrity with humor. "In our industry," he has said, "if you do a book you are legitimate and if you are on TV, you are considered a master chef."

At the taping of a celebrity chef competition in Connecticut, he arrives in a silver Lincoln with a black rag top. The camera crew has prepared two setups in the kitchen showroom studio. The first puts Ming in front of an Asian-style wood screen backdrop and a shelf holding a saki set and decanter. After a short interview taped there, he moves to a large kitchen set to chop up vegetables that will be used in the show. The crew has spent a day shooting celebrity chefs, and their energy is starting to flag. But Ming seems to bring verve onto the set: he walks in with the aura of a media professional—self-deprecating but no-nonsense. He sits down for the interview, pulls out a compact, and dabs pancake on his forehead. Clearly Ming is a media pro.

When the camera starts rolling, he's asked to describe the secret of his success. Throughout the day, the other chefs have typically invoked their passion for cooking, or their love of food. Ming is the only one to mention his family, saying he married well. He says success depends on the people you surround yourself with.

This TV kitchen studio is a long way from the shopping mall food court in Dayton where Ming's mother opened her restaurant, Mandarin Kitchen. Ming started there at fourteen and before long was working in the kitchen. His father was a mechanical and aeronautics engineer at the nearby air force base whose work often took him to Korea, and he would come home with little hospitality souvenirs, usually foil packets of ginseng tea. The ginseng was powdered or crystallized into tiny pellets, and Ming recalls the tea as a space-age fusion of East and West, combining the convenience of Tang with the complex flavor and traditional power of ginseng. When his mother brewed ginseng tea, Ming would have it too, with honey. He grew to appreciate the tannic flavor, and over time discovered new facets in it. There was the slightly mentholated aftertaste, for instance. He liked it. Most of his friends in Dayton preferred the syrupy sweetness of Coke.

Asked to share a cooking secret, Ming launches into background on his East-West approach, how he dislikes the term *fusion* because as an engineering student at Yale, for him the word meant mixing atoms, and that sounded too cold for cooking. He prefers *blending*. But to blend two cuisines, you first have to learn the traditional uses of the ingredients. How do the Chinese use sesame oil? How do Thai and Malaysian cooks use lemongrass? He mentions mango-and-pork potstickers and his love of Julia Child. The crew is rapt—he's the most charismatic talent they've had all day—but Ming catches himself. The producer wanted just twenty seconds. "You mean twenty real seconds?" he asks. "As opposed to twenty Ming Tsai seconds?"

Ming has cooked with ginseng most of his life and has a fine sense of how the root strikes different palates. At Mandarin Kitchen, the root was too expensive to add to dishes for the casual Dayton mall patron. And he wouldn't try it on patrons at Blue Ginger because they wouldn't expect it. For them, it would appear from nowhere, this tannic bitter taste that stays in the mouth. "Ginseng's not like truffles or really high-grade vanilla bean or something that will make people go, 'Wow, this is really good,'" Ming says, "because they have nothing to compare it to."

In family trips to Europe and Asia, Ming got to taste other mutations of the traditional and the modern. (In China he and his brother were shocked to be regarded as foreigners.) He found ginseng in Taiwan's Snake Alley, near Taipei, in a scene that is seared onto his brain: stall after stall of various snakes cooked alive in broth. Most of those broths included ginseng, both for culinary and for business reasons. The business reason was that high-end customers liked to combine legendary tonics, so by adding a slice of ginseng, the Alley chefs could charge substantially more for a mediocre dish.

At home, the family added ginseng to soups. Making a chicken-mushroom or an Asian-style soup, for example, Ming's mother would toss in a little root. But you had to know what it could stand up to. "Because it is a very delicate flavor," he says, "you wouldn't add it to a cream soup, for example. You'd have to use a clear broth-type soup." In general, soups are the best medium for drawing every last drop from the root and balancing it with other flavors like smoked ham or other meats. Ming would never add ginseng slices to a stir-fry, for example; even a small slice would make the dish too bitter. You need to braise the root with a nice, clear stock.

When Ming was studying engineering at Yale (he was expected to follow his father's path), he and a friend would take the train into New York's Chinatown and buy ampules of ginseng. The glass ampules came with a small, round stone that you used to file a line in the glass. Then you'd crack it open and stick a little straw into the ginseng liquid. It was an exotic technology that gave you a little kick, an energy shooter for times when you felt down. The ampules weren't expensive, and tasted surprisingly sweet. Ming would knock those shooters back, curious about the rumor that ginseng preserved youth and restored your vitality.

"I think that was what Red Bull came from," he says, in a half-joking reference to the popular energy drink. "That was my first Red Bull."

MING TIES ON A white apron at the second camera setup and flourishes his special white-bladed knife over his own cutting board. He grabs a red pepper, and as the camera rolls, he slices it lengthwise, flips it, and slices it into thin cross-sectional strips. The white blade then goes through an English cucumber in a series of incredibly fine slicing motions. The cameraman moves in for a close-up on the cucumber. When Ming finishes, the crew bursts into applause for the first time that day.

When Ming realized that he had no desire to become an engineer, a visit to a friend in Paris reawakened his love of cooking. He later returned to Paris and studied at Le Cordon Bleu, the famous French cooking school. Paris was where he discovered East-West cuisine. And there, on a third continent, he found ginseng in the city's blend of traditions and the Thirteenth Arrondisement's Chinatown. The roots were sold in stores, dried in powders and in teas, and restaurants had ginseng sprinkled among their menu items, depending on the market price and the season.

"I would bike to Chinatown, fill up my bag, and bike to Natacha," the gourmet restaurant where he was sous-chef. Ming would show the head chef what he had brought: black beans, spring-roll wrappers, wood ear mushrooms. "Ginseng," Ming says, "didn't make the bike trip."

Years later, in an inventive mood at Blue Ginger, Ming tried ginseng in a dessert. He had settled on a ginger-ginseng cake that seemed promising. When it was finished, though, he couldn't taste the ginseng. "You could taste ginger, because ginger is a stronger, fiery, spicy flavor," he told me. "But the ginseng was kind of lost." It didn't make the menu. Ginseng is too pricey to hide in the background.

For years, Ming commuted from Massachusetts to New York every few months to tape his TV series for the Food Network. He makes cooking fun as he shows how to make surprising dishes like Asian gazpacho. In one episode of *East Meets West*, he introduced viewers to his winter-melon soup, and there he tossed in some ginseng. Ming's winter-melon soup is a Shanghai-style tonic dish. You take a whole winter melon and bake it for hours. The soup forms slowly inside the melon, which you then stuff with ginger, basil, ginseng, and Chinese ham. Scrape the soup out of the melon and serve.

"It's awesome," he says. "Traditionally you would have someone carve the outside of the melon with dragons, flowers. It's phenomenal." Other ginseng dishes in his repertoire include a Beijing-style soup in which a whole duck is braised in lots of ginseng and red dates, which add a sweetness that balances the ginseng flavor.

People continue to bring new dishes and new versions of old

favorites from their travels. Ming's father doesn't hesitate to pull out a camera at a restaurant table and snap a particularly delightful winter-melon soup to e-mail his son later. Favorites include a Beijing dish of old duck, cut into chunks and seasoned with tonic herbs. In Hongzhou, the town outside Shanghai where Ming's grandmother grew up, the elder Tsais sampled a casserole of slow-cooked old duck with ham, dried bamboo shoots, and ginseng. In Seoul they tried a famous soup called Fou Tiao Chiang, or Monk Jump Wall. It comes in a covered jar and is steamed slowly, blending ham, mushrooms, chicken feet, ginseng, and more. The soup's name comes from the idea that it was so delectable—almost sexual—that monks would jump the monastery wall for it. Another photo showed Ming's mother at a famous Seoul restaurant, with a poster showing a bowl of Monk Jump Wall in the background over her shoulder.

Surprisingly, Ming has never heard of American ginseng. "I would never have known that," he says. As we talk he became more animated. He asks about how Native Americans used ginseng. And if the two species were separated by continental drift, does that mean there's an American ginger as well? Ginger is a rhizome, like ginseng. I see where this could lead. If there were a native American ginger, the name Blue Ginger could have much more resonance for East-West cuisine than he previously realized.

As it happens, there *is* a North American herb known as wild ginger *(Asarum canadense),* but it belongs to a different family than real ginger. Wild ginger smells like ginger but it's much slower growing and not a good substitute. (*Zingiber officinale,* the main ginger species, has no American cousin. It was brought from Asia to Jamaica and the West Indies by Spanish colonists centuries ago, and became a staple of Caribbean cuisine, notably ginger beer.) Ming is nevertheless intrigued. American ginseng's existence seems to open up a new facet of a familiar ingredient for him. Near the end of our talk he asks where he could get a good sample to try, so I put him in touch with Bob Beyfuss for some New York roots. Meanwhile, Ming says if I go to China, he can suggest a place that serves fantastic ginseng dishes. I accept his offer, although it's not a taste for which I would have ever predicted traveling halfway around the world.

TWELVE

Back in China

The Manchurians say that the success of the man who
starts on a perilous journey across the taiga in search of the
Root of Life depends entirely on his moral qualities.
—Nikolai Baikov, Harbin, Manchuria, 1936

Puning was the big unknown. Paul Hsu had insisted that to understand the full arc of the American ginseng trade, one had to visit China, and in particular this town on the South China coast. "To talk about ginseng, you ought to visit Puning," he said. According to him, Puning was becoming a more important distribution hub than Hong Kong, which had held the monopoly for generations. In the 1990s, as mainland China's ginseng imports grew, importers began looking for ways to bypass Hong Kong. Many of them gravitated to Puning. But Hsu was vague about how the ginseng got there.

"Under water," he deadpanned. "It's very hard to get there, you know. It's in the boondocks." He laughed. "That's the *center* in China for American ginseng."

Depending on your source, Puning had a reputation as either the smuggling capital of China or the medicinal herb capital.

Kim Wu, the Shanghai native who would be my translator there, told me by e-mail that Puning, notorious for its smuggling industry, "is the most wild place."

"All sorts of weird things happening there," Kim said, "way beyond your imagination." The BBC reported in 2001 that Puning residents had pulled the largest export tax fraud scheme ever uncovered. Local police had summarily executed four businessmen involved, but the whole area was steeped in the smuggling scandal. According to the BBC, the scam involved over a hundred criminal groups that included housewives and senior citizens, who together defrauded China's central government of almost half a billion dollars. The swindle was "an open secret in the area, with people from all walks of life becoming involved . . ."

FOR ME, TRACKING AMERICAN ginseng's reunion with its Asian roots meant following it from Hong Kong to the mainland port of Guangzhou (formerly Canton), up the coast to Puning, and further north to Nanjing.

As soon as I stepped off the plane, I felt the buzz I get from travel. In a new place the world is temporarily stripped of its everyday laminate, the sounds and smells are vivid, and I get the roller-coaster nerves of figuring out a sign or a person's gesture. First in Beijing, after gazing across the wide sea of Tiannamen Square and navigating through the impressive subway, I met Dr. Lily Sun, a family friend of Ming Tsai who invited me to lunch at Shen's Delicious Soups, a restaurant on the east side of the city. There, amid bright red décor and two rows of large pots, we enjoyed the Shanghai tradition of tonic cuisine. The row of brown pots contained "slow" soups: medicinal soups that simmered for days on gas burners. "Fast" soups, which cooked for only five or six hours, were in the row of white pots.

Lily Sun was a clinical trials manager for the international pharmaceutical firm Pharmacia. Having grown up north of Beijing and studied at Stanford, she now managed medical research throughout China, overseeing the scientific requirements of experimental design. Lily respected the diagnostic ability of the chef at Shen's Delicious Soups. One evening sometime before I arrived, she asked him which soup would help for a rash on her face. The chef recommended dishes that suited your symptoms as well as your palate, she explained. We ordered ginseng oolong tea and two entrées that contained ginseng. The first was a small portion of "herbal medicine, snake, and chicken soup," and the second was a larger dish of dark-chicken ginseng soup. The chef probably wouldn't recommend both together, but I had only one chance for a meal here, and I wanted to make the most of it.

When the dishes arrived, a slim root of fresh Asian ginseng bobbed near the surface of the dark-chicken broth. The other soup had both Asian and American ginsengs, as well as an unfamiliar, beanlike medicinal herb. Both dishes were well seasoned and flavorful, but they tasted, well, like chicken soup. The lighter soup had just a slight aftertaste, a kind of mentholation.

The ginseng taste was not meant to be a highlight, Lily explained. It was there mainly to add a healthy dimension, the idea of good health. The aftertaste proved you were getting your money's worth and a revivifying meal. We also ordered a plate of steamed greens and a shallow pan of something like stone soup. The stones were there just for heat—the dish was roast beef and scallions. It was delicious. We followed that with Shanghai-style pork dumpling, delicately cooked. But it was the mentholated chicken soup that stayed in my mouth for several hours afterward. Lily said good-bye at the subway station and wished me well. Sitting on the boxy blue Beijing subway car, I exhaled into my cupped hand, trying to savor, or at least recognize, the taste of good health.

IN HONG KONG, I walked up and down the island's steep canyons of high-rises and tried to sort out the story of American ginseng and its place here. Mainly what I wanted to know was, How did American ginseng come in and how did it go on to the mainland? Although returned to China by the British in 1997, Hong Kong retained its independent spirit, and imports that arrived duty-free there were still subject to tariffs and restrictions on the mainland. In many ways Hong Kong remained a unique place, old and new.

The Hong Kong market for American ginseng is staggering—open bins of roots, alongside umbrella mushrooms, seahorses, and other medicinals, fill nearly five full blocks of Wing Lok Street (the name means "Forever Happy") near the harbor. For over a hundred and fifty years, Chinese traders had brought traditional medicines down the Pearl River and traded them in Hong Kong's free port. The city's yellow pages had two headings dedicated to ginseng: Ginseng Products & Herbs, Retailers (286 listings); and Ginseng Products & Herbs, Wholesalers (105 listings). And that was just the English-language edition.

I walked down to the docks and stepped aboard the green ferryboat that crossed the harbor in the morning, where the crew wore blue sailor outfits with stars on their kerchiefs. As I watched a barge pass near us, loaded with red shipping containers and rimmed with tractor tires hanging off its sides, I tried to reconcile conflicting reports. A CITES official on the Kowloon side of the harbor told me that she expected that in the future American ginseng shipments would bypass Hong Kong and go straight to mainland ports, but she hadn't seen that shift yet. Paul Hsu had indicated that the shift had already happened. There also appeared to be a disconnect between the official figures for incoming and outgoing American ginseng: officially, that year Hong Kong imported 4,583,812 kilograms and exported 3,008,205 kilograms. That would mean that local consumers bought over 1,575,600 kilograms of American ginseng roots, which translated to about a half pound for every man, woman, and child in Hong Kong.

I understood that local demand was high. (According to Hong Kong *Tatler* that month, the island's traditional medicine sector had grown by 10 percent in three years, fueled by the emotional stress of a depressed economy and its effects on the island's stockbrokers. An epidemic of impotence was traced to the stresses of financial woes, depression, and "damp-heat" infections, and ginseng was a popular remedy, along with antler velvet and deer penis, dried seahorses, and an herb known as Horny Goat Weed.) Still, half a pound per person? It seemed more likely that a lot of ginseng was being exported under the radar.

I stopped in a bare-bones shop on Wing Lok Street and looked into the open wooden bins. The clerk offered me a sample of what she said was good-quality ginseng: HK$330 per tael (the traditional unit of measure), or US$920 a pound. Using paring shears, she shaved off two samples and I popped them in my mouth.

"Wisconsin," she said.

Several blocks away, on the modern thoroughfare of Queens Road, red double-decker trams streamed past the chrome façade of a Madison Avenue version of the traditional medicine shop. The storefront had an emblazoned gold column and a knight in full armor, mounted on a horse. Display shelves featured pharmaceutically packaged qi pills and deer's-tail pills. In silver-fronted cases under the glass counter were squared bins of ginseng root, sorted by category: Wild American ginseng, Round-shaped, No. 4, went for about US$4,183 per pound. The expensive stuff was a package of five luxuriously long roots, Wild American No. 1 size, list price HK$120,000 — over US$3,150 per individual root. That was ten times more than I had imagined! At the low end were small packets of cultivated ginseng, sliced. I walked out with one that cost about US$11.50.

Wing Lok Street was the place to be. Paul Hsu's franchise was at one end, and Sun Ming Hong, David Law's company, was near the other end, in a building with a big Canadian maple leaf on one side. The side street resounded with a twittering of birds, which emanated from an open second-floor apartment where at least a dozen reed cages hung from the ceiling. Two shops that sold fishing tackle made a strange sight, packed among the city's offices and restaurants. It was hard to imagine fishermen among the stock traders who lived up in the Mid Levels.

Sun Ming Hong's manager, Michael Chan, opened a locked

grate and let me inside the warehouse office. Over cups of ginseng tea we sat at a bare table near a stack of boxes. He wouldn't
say exactly how much American ginseng they imported during
the previous year, but admitted he was among the top five importers. He laughed at my attempts to get more specific. "I don't
want to confirm or deny," he said.

He described the process instead. The wild ginseng that
David Law and I escorted to JFK had come into the Hong
Kong airport and was met by Chan. The law required him to
ask government CITES inspectors to check the paperwork before they could release it from the airport. After that it got ware-
housed and sold to buyers in the ginseng graders' guild. Sales
took place in two ways: through closed auctions and direct sales.
In a direct sale, Sun Ming Hong invited a buyer from within the
guild for a private showing, and there they would negotiate a
price one-on-one. The auctions were also restricted to guild
members and took place at a warehouse on Bonham Strand
near the docks. In recent years the number of auctions had declined as buyers came to prefer direct sales. Following the 2002
autumn harvest, there were only three auctions near the New
Year celebration. Sun Ming Hong's was the last.

At the auction, the importer poured out the barrels of roots
onto a mat, and buyers would inspect and mentally grade the
lot. They would calculate, on the computer in their head, *If I set
this crop price with these different classifications, approximately
how much money is this batch worth?* They would write a figure
on a slip of paper, and Sun Ming Hong would collect the bids
and accept the highest offer. The drums would be resealed by a
guild official, who would then write on it the name of the

buyer. The buyer could then either take the CITES paperwork and reexport the lot, or sell that ginseng within Hong Kong.

Sun Ming Hong worked mainly through the guild, as it has for over a half century. David Law and Chan both had relatives in the ginseng business, and their families had known each other since they were kids. Chan had gone to Australia and studied electrical engineering, never intending to join the family business. Like Law, he was trained as a scientist but nonetheless believed in the empirical evidence of Chinese clinical experience.

"Chinese look at ginseng as what we call a catalyst to improve your health," he said, not as a drug that directly improves health. He understood the Western scientific search to find agents that directly cause a physiological change, but said it's just not that easy with herbs in Chinese medicine. He drew an analogy from chemistry to explain the use of American ginseng and Asian ginseng. If a pH of 7 (that is, neutral) were the norm, then you would want to balance your body pH close to 7. How you get there depends on your starting point: some people are more acidic, so they would want to raise their level; others who are more alkaline would want to lower it. Based on an individual's system, you would prescribe Asian ginseng or American ginseng. This analogy fit reasonably well with what pharmacologist Varro Tyler had said: "If you're overwrought and you want to take ginseng to calm down a little bit, American ginseng may be your herb of choice. If you need energy to pep up and so on, then the Asian ginseng would be the herb of choice."

The business had changed a lot since the 1960s, when the American ginseng market was controlled by a small group in

New York. "I should not use the word *mafia,*" Chan said. "New York traders, cartel, whatever. Monopolistic traders." The cartel kept Sun Ming Hong from buying directly from Appalachian harvesters. Only in the 1970s, when David Law began his road trips, did the company manage to bypass the cartel and deal directly between American diggers and wholesale buyers in Asia.

Chan was vague about ongoing changes in the industry but admitted that his business model was conservative. "Perception and reputation, to me, are more important than making some money," he said. Yes, the business was shifting to the mainland, but he couldn't really say where. He left that to others. In eight years he had seen demand on the mainland increase tremendously, mainly for cheaper cultivated roots. But mainland policy changes were confusing, and he was frustrated by the growing bureaucracy around ginseng.

IN CONTRAST WITH Sun Ming Hong's warehouse, Hsu's Root to Health was a small retail shop open at street level. When the branch manager, Simon Wong, came forward from the back room, I was startled by his youth. We sat before the counter and chatted, his knee bouncing with energy the whole time. Behind the counter his two clerks measured out the daily special of dried plants into plastic packets, and served the occasional customer.

The differences between the two operations were stark. If Sun Ming Hong was an old-school wholesale importer, Hsu's company was a modern, aggressively integrated corporation. Hsu had expanded vertically, from farm source to retailer, and then horizontally, widening his range of products beyond ginseng to other medicinals. "Our trading method is an enterprising one," said Wong approvingly.

Wong had no family connections in the ginseng business. When he was a kid, ginseng was too pricey for his family. "It's kind of expensive stuff," he said. He didn't even *see* ginseng until he worked at a Hong Kong guesthouse, where Korean customers occasionally gave ginseng as gifts to his boss. Wong studied journalism in Texas and moved to New York, where he took a job as a reporter for a Chinese-language paper in Chinatown. He met Paul Hsu there in 1994, and soon began working in Hsu's New York branch. After a year Wong returned to Hong Kong to help launch a new branch of Hsu's.

When the Asian financial crisis struck in 1997, imports of wild American ginseng slumped drastically. Just as Wong was getting his feet on the ground with the new store on the Kowloon side of the harbor, the region's economy bottomed out. The main branch manager quit, and Wong, who had expected to be learning one shop as a deputy, found himself running both branches.

With the economy still down, Wong's customers wanted the cheap cultivated roots that came by surface, along with things like birds' nests. He handled e-mail, faxes, and phone calls about shipments all over Asia. (Most customers still preferred to send orders by fax, not e-mail, because so many Chinese characters couldn't be entered on a computer keyboard. For tracking shipments, e-mail worked fine.) Just measuring orders required another wizardry of translation: American Chinese use ounces; Hong Kong uses the traditional units of taels and cattys that date back to the Qing era; and mainland consumers use grams. When a ship came in, Wong would send a truck to the Kowloon shipping terminals and ask CITES officials to certify the cargo for release. "They need to chop," he said, punching his knee in a stamping motion. I imagined the square, red-inked stamp coming down—the same type of chop that the *Empress of China* needed in order to dock in Canton. The CITES office would send over an official who opened drums randomly, maybe one in ten, for inspection.

As a former journalist, Wong empathized with my effort to get a full panorama of the ginseng story, when people only wanted to show narrow slices of the landscape. He offered help with the Hong Kong ginseng graders' guild, Po Sau Tong, but cautioned it was a tight, secret society and only one or two members might talk with me. He introduced me to a member he called Sister Lin, who managed a shop on Queens Road West and dealt almost exclusively in ginseng. We found the place off an alley. Dozens of open bins with different-shaped roots stretched into her shop, behind displays of dried sea cucumber. At the entrance stood a small red offering to the spirits, and a banner overhead trumpeted the Wisconsin Ginseng Board. On the wall hung a cherished package of rare wild Asian ginseng, retail price about US$1,200. Wild American roots in the bins, wild Asian roots on the wall. Here was where the two ginsengs had their reunion—not in a shady, mixed mesophytic forest, but in this bustling urban marketplace.

Choi Oi Lin had a good smile. She had worked in the industry for over twenty years and was one of just a handful of women who had risen within the graders' guild. Unlike the other women, who had a husband or a brother in the business, Lin had no family connections. She claimed modestly that she was still learning about the various grades of roots, but she showed me how her graders spot fine differences. She looks at a root's color, shape, wrinkle, size, and texture. How does it feel between the fingers? She could tell American ginseng grown in China from the same species grown in America.

"American-grown is slightly more dense than China-grown," she said. Wild ginseng is harder to grade than cultivated because there are twice as many categories (over fifty), and because there's more at stake: price differences among the grades are steeper than between grades of cultivated root. Again, graders have to master regional preferences: buyers in Hong Kong and Guangzhou want to see the neck scars, but others cut the neck off. Lin's graders used hand shears to trim and sort the roots into different categories. The trimmings made a further category. After a while she excused herself; business was pressing.

Things were much quieter at the legendary guild office, Po Sau Tong Ginseng & Antler Association. The big silver characters dominated a dim elevator lobby on the second floor of a nondescript commercial building. The door was locked, so I rang the bell. I could see a light on inside, and beyond, the conference room shades were drawn. Nobody answered. The place was a sanctuary of silence amid the noisy streets.

A SHORT TRAIN RIDE from Hong Kong, Guangzhou was a rainy boomtown, old and new at once, sprawling across the Pearl River. There you could glimpse the retail side of the ginseng industry in the Xingping market. Xingping, one of the first markets in the country that opened for business in the late 1970s under Deng Xiaoping's market reforms, was a warren of walkways and covered one-room shop stalls. It stood opposite the old foreigner district where European sailors and merchants were housed in the 1700s.

In the market I followed my translator, Raymond (the name he asked me to call him, to save me from mangling his real name), past rows and rows of herb dealers. Sacks full of ginseng slices stood alongside boxes of umbrella mushrooms and sea horses. This was Home Depot–style medicine. Nobody came here to fill a doctor's Rx or an herbalist's scrip; there were pharmacies for that. This was discount stuff. As we threaded past stall after stall, Raymond explained that he never bought ginseng sliced because he suspected that sellers would have sucked out all the extract. He preferred to buy whole roots.

We spoke with a ginseng dealer in his twenties who had a certain *yakuza*-like style, with his buttoned dark blue suit and no tie. He grew up in Puning and had started as a ginseng grader, and now trucked American roots down the coast four hundred kilometers to the market. He apparently thought I was an exporter looking for a way to sell my roots sub rosa in the Chinese market, just as American merchants had trawled the Canton shops in the eighteenth century, looking for black market openings.

My efforts to find the landing point of the *Empress of China* began with promise. Raymond found the street that was once home to the Co Hong merchants' guild: Shi Sang Hang Lu, or "Thirteen Companies Street." Then he led the way to the harbor and Huangpu (or Whampoa) Island, where the *Empress* had docked for her customs chop over two hundred years before. The place turned out to be an industrial desert. Guangzhou's explosive growth was obliterating even newer homes while people still lived in them. There was little hope of finding the nine-story pagoda that loomed over the harbor two centuries ago, but I insisted we try.

After asking directions several times, we came to an ancient-looking pagoda that rose above a disheveled garden. In a quagmire nearby, a dragon boat lay on its side. A woman working in a nearby factory said that more likely we were looking for the taller pagoda that was destroyed during the Cultural Revolution.

RAYMOND WARNED THAT THE road to Puning was risky. There were smugglers up the coast who could be dangerous, he said. He laughed at the insanity of taking a bus, and urged me to keep some money in my wallet for handing over to thieves so they would leave satisfied. The rest I should hide against my chest.

I considered his advice on the bus as *Rumble in the Bronx* played on the screen above the driver's head. Outside my window the craggy and undulating peaks looked fantastic, like the brushstrokes of a Chinese painting. The bus left the highway amid more swooping mountains and took a road into Puning that was wide and rough. We entered town on a commercial strip with shop after shop of wholesale items for which I couldn't imagine any local demand: a load of brand new minivans still in their shipping plastic, acetylene torches, shops full of plumbing fixtures. The place itself appeared to be undergoing great changes, but it was impossible to tell if it was explosive growth or explosive demolition. Whole city blocks were covered in rubble, studded with ruins, and people were walking over the debris like war survivors. We passed stacks of huge tires, a cannibalized truck. A stagnant river.

The driver caught my eye in the rearview mirror and shot his right arm out, indicating my hotel as we passed. It was the only hotel licensed to handle foreigners (I didn't see another non-Chinese during my entire stay). That evening I met Kim, my translator, a diminutive woman in a wool plaid jacket that she wore the whole time I knew her. She explained that Puning had been a smuggling center ever since China began opening up under Deng Xiaoping in 1979. It started with small electronics and quickly scaled up to cars and larger goods. Local officials saw an unlocked door and they opened it. But people were reluctant to talk. Apparently the murdered businessmen mentioned in the BBC report I read had been invited by Beijing, so their deaths at the hands of local police drew the central government's wrath. More recently, a smuggling case in Xiamen up the coast diverted the spotlight from Puning, but the town was still under central government surveillance, Kim said. People here were terrified of drawing more attention. We really didn't know what sort of reception we would get from Hsu's colleague Xu Wei Ming the next morning, or what kind of conversation we would have.

I LOWERED MY HOPES for learning anything in Puning. The morning after I arrived, a dark green sedan with curtained back windows pulled in front of the hotel, and Xu Wei Ming stepped out. Xu (pronounced like *shoe*) was a nimble man, younger than I expected. He was dressed in a less formal version of the business-cum-*yakuza* fashion preferred by the young men on Puning's streets: a dark sweater with a sportcoat and dark slacks, tan loafers. On his lapel he wore a red-and-blue button for Paul Hsu's Root to Health. He was slim, about forty years old, and walked with his head high, looking friendly but preoccupied.

Xu was eager to show off the medicinal herb complex that had put Puning on the map. Puning's position between the mountains and the sea, he explained, was key to the town's traditions in herbal medicine. Puning had a local expertise that was generations old but had mushroomed in economic importance in two decades. Guangzhou's Xingping market might have been the first to open after Deng's reforms, but Puning was among the first to take advantage of the scope for growth. The Puning government, anxious to court business, helped the town's medicinal herb dealers eclipse the Guangzhou market by putting up money to build the market complex and by declining to collect import tariffs imposed by the central government. Smuggling was therefore a rather crude term for what the locals preferred to call a policy of local economic empowerment.

When Xu shows visitors around the herb market complex, he speaks of its hardware in a way that can be confusing until you know that people in China like to use the word *hardware* whenever possible. Xu himself entered the medicinal herb business when he was still a teenager, over twenty years before. He grew up in a rural home, the youngest of eight children, and left school at seventeen. The medicinal herb trade then was dangerous—at that time, in the mid-1970s, *any* business enterprise in China was risky business: capitalist forays were strictly illegal. "Business was banned," Xu said, "but if you were bold enough, you could make good money." He dug the herbs himself, gradually putting together a stake for business. When he started, he didn't know the plants well—didn't know what he was looking for—so he asked help from the family's doctor. Xu ventured deeper into remote areas, bought herbs from villagers, and sold them in town.

He was barely twenty years old when he had amassed enough money to build an expensive house for his parents. In China building a house is more than a way to show status—it's a duty to show that each generation is doing better than the one before. The house Xu built for his parents stood just east of town at the foot of a mountain, facing a river in the distance. He chose the site carefully for its feng shui: having a mountain at your back and water before you is auspicious. The house is a shrine to both his family and fine craftsmanship. The carvings on the doors, the carved stone downspouts, and the undulating roofline, a *chaosan* style known as Tiger Coming Down the Mountain, all bumped the cost up to 200,000 Yuan—roughly US$25,000—a huge sum even now. (Recent government housing policy frowns on this traditional architecture, since hundreds of one-story houses use space less efficiently than a squared-off apartment building. Fewer and fewer applications to build traditional homes are being granted.)

Xu made a specialty of handling ginseng and found a niche bringing in American ginseng. He reasoned that it was worth a risk. In the same way that the government had changed its mind

and legalized local business under Deng Xiaoping twenty years
before, it might eventually legalize the international black market that skirted the current tariff on foreign goods. In other
words, if the experience with market reform was any indication,
then Xu couldn't afford *not* to get involved in smuggling. If he
waited until the trade was legal, the big guys would already have
divided up the pie.

Far from being a nest of cramped stalls like the market in
Guangzhou, Puning's herb complex was huge and modern: a
massive gateway in front stands five stories high, and the whole
chrome-and-tinted-glass affair echoed traditional *chaosan* archi-
tecture with its winged corners and green-tiled roof. The place
resembled nothing so much as an open-air version of the Mall
of America. (At over 117 acres, the market covers an area half
again the size of the Mall of America.) It had orderly rows of
328 stucco-walled shops and a central facility that doubled as a
medicinal laboratory and stock exchange. The shop spaces had
filled quickly, each rented out on a fifty-year lease, and there
were enough wholesalers on a waiting list to warrant expanding the market's eastern flank. Many of the merchants had three
generations of experience and investment, and most were from
Puning.

The breathtaking scale of the market was the brainchild of
Chen De Feng, an herb dealer who came back from retirement
and led the effort to build the complex in 1997 with 150 million
Yuan (about $18.7 million) from the provincial government.
Chen resembles an Asian Ernest Borgnine, but better looking.
Xu compared him to Li Shizhen, the Ming-era physician whose
statue stands in front of the complex, saying his friend would

be similarly memorialized one day. (Li is the epic figure in Chinese medicine whose massive pharmocopoeia, the product of twenty-seven years of work and travel, was published in 1596.) The older man shrugged off this flattery and led us on a tour through the central building's marble halls. Chen showed off a lab for chemical analysis on the fifth floor, where a photospectrometer and other high-tech equipment waited under plastic blankets for plant samples to test. One floor below were conference rooms and meeting areas where trade and government representatives from a dozen countries had recently visited, and room after room of display cases with botanical specimens, plant exudates, mineral crystals, and animal parts. American ginseng had its own place of honor.

The Puning market's volume had tripled in less than a decade, according to Chen. He paused to point out a row of six computer monitors that tracked market prices and trends. This place set a gauge for herb prices throughout China, he said, the Dow Jones of the medicinal market. Puning was the largest hub for traditional Chinese medicine in Guangdong Province, and probably in the country. American ginseng held a small but formidable position in that market. Roots arrived in shipping containers to the port of Shantou, two hours east, and were trucked to Puning. Strolling through the market, we passed containers fitted on the back of small trucks. A series of familiar hundred-pound brown drums rolled off one container, and Xu explained that a shipment from Canada had just arrived.

At Xu's own shop, the words AMERICAN GINSENG rose above the door in gilt letters on a green background. A mural covering the left wall featured a lush green ginseng garden in Wisconsin, red berries, and the Wisconsin Ginseng Board's seal prominently displayed. And there on the end of the mural was Paul Hsu, looking prosperous and bigger than life, holding an enormous ginseng root. There was also a prominent framed photo of Hsu with President George W. Bush. Hsu has contacts within both political parties and here was the payoff: in China, a picture is worth a thousand characters for establishing authority.

Upstairs Xu described how he met Paul Hsu. (Written in Chinese characters, the two men have the same family name; they are essentially relatives whose relationship is masked by accidents of history and different transliteration systems.) In 1990 Xu was visiting Hong Kong to order a shipment of roots, and Paul Hsu was there trying to get a branch started. They connected through a mutual acquaintance, and before long Xu was buying from Hsu's Ginseng. The network of Hsu's branch offices in China (he had three, plus a headquarters in Nanjing) has made it easier to move American ginseng. Xu no longer had to travel to Hong Kong so often. Since the previous November, he told me, he had brought in more than 136,000 kilograms of root.

Xu kept pouring cups of traditional kung-fu tea for us from a small clay pot. He explained that people in Guangdong would often have tea four or five times a day, especially after meals. "Tea three, drink four" was a local saying. Its meaning escaped me completely.

We were joined by the head of the local tax collection office, a loose-limbed man in another navy blazer, who had the casual authority you might expect of a smuggler. He was affable but brusque. He interrupted to have a word with Xu over several packages of Wisconsin root and then he left. When he reappeared several times over my three days in Puning, I began to wonder if he was checking on me. At one point he noted that Puning's seafood market was a good example of how enterprising this part of Guangdong was: fishmongers came from as far as Singapore to sell their goods in Puning's market, starting at six a.m. each day; by ten a.m. everything was sold out. Puning wasn't even a major city, or on the water! It was a tribute to the people of Guangdong and their business acumen, he said.

Asked about the smuggling bust of two years before, Xu admitted that the case hurt the herb market's growth and forced dealers to pay higher taxes. The tax man tapped Xu's leg and added that it wasn't just the herb market that suffered—the whole city had been set back ten years. The municipal government had nearly gone bankrupt from it. Even worse than the central tax hike, though, was the damage to their reputation. It would take years to recover, but he was confident that Puning would rebound.

Xu added quietly that the future depended on hard work. It was encouraging that the national import tariff had dropped from 35 percent to 11 percent since China joined the WTO, and was supposed to drop further. Eventually the tariff would be so low it wouldn't be a problem. For that reason, both Xu and the taxman were pleased with globalization. Puning had eclipsed Hong Kong as a ginseng market, and now the world would follow Puning's lead.

Xu and Chen took me for seafood, a local specialty. I have never seen so many tanks of live shrimp, crabs, fish, eels, and other aquatic life. Chen pointed out the health benefits of each.

Then, over fried tofu, tender squid, fish balls, cracked crab legs and roe, skewered shrimp, and sticky-rice sweets, they complained about the capital. Beijing is so crowded, you can only get one thing done per day, they said.

"In Beijing, you realize how small an official you are," Chen said, referring to that city's concentration of high officials. He added, "In Guangdong, you realize how poor you are," a nod to the freewheeling wealth of the province's businessmen.

"And in Hainan Island, you realize how weak you are," joked Xu as he ladled out soup—a reference to the swarms of prostitutes on the resort off the Guangdong coast.

THROUGHOUT MY VISIT I was escorted from one sight to the next, treated by my hosts with great hospitality. That night in the Gold Leaf Hotel, our entourage of six or seven was ushered to a private dining/karaoke suite equipped with a full sound system and color-gel light displays. Xu and I sat on a plush sofa while the tax man stood and held forth on local politics. He talked more loudly now and seemed to be a little drunk, but during dinner he declined beer, choosing a medicinal tea instead.

Xu and I toasted each other frequently with Tsing Tao beer, and the young waitresses in red uniforms brought out dish after dish: pig's tail, fried bee larvae (light and slightly sweet), a fish-and-sweet-potato dish, apricot soup, a plate of ginger, beef, greens with pickled carrot, vegetable dumplings, more fried tofu, and very fine, delicious hand-made wheat-flour noodles. Instead of being whacked by smuggling gangs for asking pesky questions, I was being wined and dined. Cell phones jingled around the table as the lazy Susan turned. The Wisconsin farmer's comment comparing smugglers and writers came back to me. I looked around the table and thought, *It's a strange world.*

THE LAST MORNING IN Puning I dropped by Xu's store to say good-bye. He was in his office talking with a younger man from Shantou who had come to talk ginseng. On the table lay a local newspaper clipping, about new rules for money laundering. Throughout my visit to China the English-language press was full of official posturing on how corruption would no longer be tolerated.

Xu drove me and Kim back to the hotel as a farewell gesture. Passing the city's garment market he said, "Five or six years ago, you could get every kind of fabric from anywhere in the world." Now the market was nearly empty; rows and rows of traders but no business. The crackdown after the tax fraud scandal had chased business away to Guangzhou. The cigarette market was down, too. Only the herbal medicine market was left and, Xu maintained, there was never a lot of ginseng smuggled anyway. He ventured to add that whatever else smuggling did, it benefited local economies. Import tariffs, on the other hand, only helped the central government that collected them. In his view, smuggling was simply sound local policy.

EVERYWHERE YOU TURN IN China, there's a landmark that throws the past up against the present and future. In looking for ginseng's past, it was probably inevitable that I would brush up against its future. On my last day in Hong Kong, gliding along the long multiblock escalator up the mountainside to the

Mid Levels, I kept thinking about something that the Sun Ming Hong manager had said. Over cups of ginseng tea, I had asked him about the prospects for wild ginseng.

"I do not have a crystal ball for the supply of wild ginseng," he said. Then he leaned forward on one arm, his face twisted in a laugh-grimace. He said that American ginseng had a future, even if wild ginseng did not.

Looking down on the narrow streets beneath the escalator, I wondered what that meant. Maybe this was the moment in history when a plant passed the threshold from wild to wholly domesticated, beyond which it no longer had a destiny separate from people. Maybe ginseng still had a long future ahead, but without all of its mystery. Or perhaps the root's curious ability to remain dormant in the soil for years, in a sort of suspended animation, gave wild ginseng an escape hatch from the immediate pressures of extinction that other species simply didn't have. Ginseng could wait out an intense burst of digging, or a clearcut, or a flood—at least for a few years.

High on the slope above Wing Lok Street, overlooking the harbor and the Kowloon peninsula beyond, is the campus of the University of Hong Kong, with its shiny biological sciences building. My appointment to talk ginseng was not in the botany department but in the zoology lab, of course. Even in Hong Kong ginseng was wildlife. A class had just let out, releasing students wearing trendy warm-up jackets with BIOTECH-NOLOGY printed in red letters. In an office packed with an eclectic array of books—*Fish of Rare Breeding, The Evaluation of Forensic DNA Evidence, Avian Pathology*—Dr. Fred Leung told me about the future of ginseng.

Leung spoke about it in the terms of Chinese medicine—of hot and cold—but he could also discuss ginsenoside content and the results of clinical trials. He had worked in the United States for years at Merck, the pharmaceutical giant. "I think genetics will tell the truth of who you are," he said. "When I look at Chinese herbal medicine, my culture tells me, 'Yeah it works,' but my scientific background says, 'I lack data.' So that's where I got into looking at the genetics of herbs."

He invented a method for "fingerprinting" ginseng using its DNA sequences. For that, he extracted DNA by grinding dried roots to a fine powder in liquid nitrogen, adding an extraction solution, and incubating the mixture for half an hour. After cooling and further extraction, he put the solution in a centrifuge and out came a DNA pellet. With that he identified a gene sequence that occurred repeatedly, in both *Panax* species. Because the sequence was four to five times more abundant in Asian ginseng, it gave him an easy method for identifying, from a tiny sample, whether a root was Asian or American ginseng. A DNA library of ginseng genomic variation helped him to find other identification markers for distinguishing smaller differences. Leung's fingerprinting technique does what graders in Hong Kong say they do based on color, texture, and shape: determine where the plant comes from and compare it with others. As a result, Wisconsin farmers have buttonholed Leung at meetings and asked him to fingerprint their ginseng's DNA so they could prove its provenance. He said he can distinguish Wisconsin ginseng from New York ginseng, and even one farm's ginseng from another ten miles away. This capability could authenticate marketing claims and also reveal the original sources of seed material. Paul Hsu said of Leung's work, "I can tell the root from the outside, he can tell it from the inside." Besides confirming a root's source, Leung hoped that his work could serve the medical community and eventually provide a profile of the plant's bio-efficacy against human ailments. That was a long shot, but if successful, it might go a long way to change the perceptions of Western consumers.

Merchants, however, weren't interested. In Asia, where the biggest market was, you didn't need science to sell ginseng; you just needed the supply. People there already believed in ginseng, and more information did not necessarily pay off. "That whole marketing scheme is unbelievable," Leung said. He pointed down the hill. "There is more ginseng right now in Kennedy Town warehouses than in the rest of the world."

Ginseng's journey always points to surprising connections, but like Leung's research, it also points to gaps in understanding. People who buy wild ginseng are usually unaware of their link to forests in America and the health of those forests. And nobody yet knows exactly what happens when a medicinal herb enters the human body. Burrowing into ginseng's genetic makeup might answer some questions even as it raises others.

Leung expected that the industry would eventually adopt a standard technique for identifying roots and their genetic sources. I thought of all the human fingerprints on the ginseng pouring into Hong Kong's warehouses, and the stories and tangled strands of traditions that came with them: Jerry Wolf's roots from Cherokee, Jeanine Davis's farmers' plants in western Carolina, Fred Hays's simulated-wild root from the Kanawha Valley, Abraham Yi Vang and his farm's produce in central Wisconsin. The roots under the white tents of Bob Beyfuss's Catskill ginseng festival, all moving as fast as they could toward people with low qi. Despite warnings of its demise, ginseng still seemed to have a lot of energy and mystique left in it.

At least some of the mystery that people attributed to ginseng came from within themselves, I realized. It was a *Wizard of Oz* moment: the scene where the wizard observes that the scarecrow already has a brain, and Dorothy has been carrying her home within her all along. With ginseng Nurhaci had summoned the power of the Manchus, and Lafitau had detected a key to his theory of relations between the Old and New Worlds. Bob Beyfuss found in it a channel for his own energy and efforts in conservation. The answer to ginseng's future in the wild, how it gains and loses value, the puzzle of its chemical interactions—all these were inseparable from people. "It certainly is closely tied to humans," Gary Kauffman, the Forest Service botanist, had said. "Maybe to its detriment."

This close relationship might suggest something else, too. In searching for ginseng's secrets, we glimpse what we value as humans. Its history tells us how much people through the ages have treasured good food, good health, and wealth, but also intangibles like tradition, longevity, and even (very recently) biodiversity. People are ginseng's predators, its dispersal agents, and in rare cases, its protectors. Right now the plant is poised at a precarious junction. In the end, we will probably grasp ginseng's true nature only when we appreciate our own mysterious place in the natural world.

ACKNOWLEDGMENTS

MANY PEOPLE HELPED to make this book, from start to finish.
Most of those who generously gave their time and experience
appear in the list of sources. Bob Beyfuss, Dave Cooke, Paul
Hsu, and David Law were especially helpful. Lamon Brown,
Randy Brunn, Jim Corbin, Jeanine Davis, Susan Eng, Jim
Garrison, Fred Hays, Ming Tsai, Abraham Yi Vang, and Jerry
Wolf also provided important insights for understanding ginseng and its path. Christopher Robbins, of TRAFFIC International, and Phoebe Sze, of the CITES Management Authority
in Hong Kong, answered a stream of questions with good humor. William Lass, Andreas Motsch, and Van Symons provided
important historical information. Burkhard Bilger and W. Scott
Persons were also generous with their time and expertise.

William Clark, my agent, believed in this book from the start
and pointed the way. Antonia Fusco, my editor at Algonquin,
gave invaluable guidance, support, and encouragement. This
would not have happened without their enthusiasm.

In China, I owe much to the hospitality of Xu Wei Ming in
Puning, Dr. Lily Sun in Beijing, and Simon Wong and Michael

Chan in Hong Kong. I would also like to thank my translator-guides: Luo Zheng in Guangzhou, Kim Wu in Puning, Sun Jun in Nanjing, and Jia Suang Fang in Shenyang.

I'm grateful to Kate Blackwell, Stephanie Joyce, Gary Kauffman, and John F. Ross for offering important suggestions and comments on various drafts, and to my family for their constant support. Above all, Lisa Smith gave me her priceless editorial eye, along with her endless support, patience, insight, and love.

Ginseng Use and Recipes

THERE ARE SEVERAL WAYS to take ginseng root as a simple tonic, besides the many packaged products that list ginseng as an ingredient. This section is not a prescription, however. Before using ginseng or any other medicinal herb, you should consult a certified herbalist, a nutritionist, and/or your physician.

When buying dried ginseng, choose firm, light-colored roots and avoid shriveled ones. Roots usually come washed and dried. You can store them in a sealed plastic bag in your refrigerator's crisper for up to ten days. In his book *American Ginseng: Green Gold*, Scott Persons notes that the optimal daily dose is 2–3 grams per day—roughly equivalent to a section of dried root about the size of an almond sliver or your little fingernail.

The two most common ways to prepare ginseng are as chewable root slices or as tea. Dried root slices can be chewed like a kind of licorice or jerky. For a pot of ginseng tea, place a dozen or so thin root slices in about a quart of boiling water, using more hot water as needed. People often add honey or sugar to improve the taste.

A third way to prepare ginseng is to place a sliver of root in a broth-style soup and let it simmer for an hour or so (see below). For ginseng-flavored honey, place a whole, washed root in a honey jar. You can make a stronger concoction by placing a slim, whole fresh root in a bottle of vodka.

In traditional Chinese medicine, ginseng is part of a balanced diet that is based not on food groups but on yin and yang (see chapter 11). In this view, everything—and everyone—consists, to varying degrees, of yin and yang. What constitutes a balanced diet depends on whether a person is predominantly yin or predominantly yang. People who are more yang are often outgoing, sometimes aggressive, and more likely to feel warm and to suffer from stress, congestion, constipation, headaches, heart disease, and other yang-type illnesses, according to Dr. Maoshing Ni, quoted in *New Choices in Natural Healing for Women* by Barbara Loecher. Yin people, on the other hand, tend to be calm and reflective, sensitive to cold, and more vulnerable to fatigue, obesity, and diarrhea.

Foods that have a warming effect, such as chili peppers, are mostly yang. Watermelon and other foods that cool the body are mostly yin. Asian ginseng is said to be yang; American ginseng, yin. There are also neutral foods, such as brown rice and lettuce, that neither warm nor cool the body. A healthy diet includes all three types in balanced proportions. "Generally speaking, such a diet is heavy on grains and vegetables; uses a lot of beans and soy products; includes some fruits, nuts and seeds; and uses protein, like red meat, poultry and fish, as a condiment," says Dr. Ni. The menu also changes with the seasons.

Here are a few recipes from several different sources. To prepare the roots for cooking, remove all dirt and place them in water for about ten minutes. Scrub off the remaining dirt with a small brush under running water. Some sources suggest trimming off the minor forks, sometimes called "fine ginseng," as they can taste more bitter than the rest of the root.

GINSENG AND CHICKEN CASSEROLE

1 whole chicken
12 slices yam, peeled
2 tablespoons whole Chinese wolfberries
1 medium-size piece ginseng
2 slices ginger, peeled
1 spring onion, cut into lengths
6 cups chicken broth
1 teaspoon salt
¼ cup rice wine
8 mushrooms

Cut the whole chicken down its back and place in boiling water for 2–3 minutes, then wash the chicken in cold water. Put the yam slices, wolfberries, and ginseng into a stewing pan and place the chicken on top of them. Add the ginger and onion. Pour the broth in, add the rice wine and salt, and cover the pan tightly; let the mixture simmer at a low heat for about 2 hours. Soak the mushrooms in warm water. Add them and stew for 1 hour more. Remove the ginger and onion. Place the ginseng on the chicken and serve. Makes 6–8 servings.

Adapted from www.China-on-site.com.

GINSENG AND BEEF

    1 tablespoon soy sauce

    1 tablespoon wine or sherry

    ½ teaspoon sugar

    ½ pound tenderloin, cut into narrow strips
       or chunks

    3 cloves garlic, finely chopped

    Vegetable oil

    Up to ½ cup ginseng root, fresh or
       dried, thoroughly cleaned and thinly sliced

    ⅛ teaspoon ground black pepper

    3–4 scallions

Mix together the soy sauce, sherry, and sugar. Marinate the beef in the soy sauce mixture in a bowl; cover and refrigerate for 2 hours. Remove the meat and reserve the marinade. Stir-fry the garlic and meat in oil until cooked through. Add the ginseng and sauté briefly while adding the soy sauce marinade and pepper to taste. Add the scallions and cook for 1-2 minutes. Makes 4–6 servings.

Adapted from www.hsuginseng.com.

WINTER-MELON SOUP

2 pounds winter melon (*dong gua,* a melon with pale,
   sweet flesh found in Asian groceries)
1 teaspoon salt
6 cups chicken stock
1 small ginseng root
4 ounces straw mushrooms
⅓ cup shredded, cooked chicken breast
2 slices fresh ginger, peeled
¼ cup cooked or canned crabmeat
¼ cup canned asparagus tips, drained
6 dried lotus nuts, soaked and peeled,
   with the hard core removed
Cilantro leaves

Look for a winter melon that will hold at least 6 cups of liquid. Cut off the top. (If the melon is very large, slice it in half so that half will hold the soup.) Remove the melon's central fiber and seeds. Scrape out some of the flesh, leaving a layer about 3/4-inch thick still clinging to the inside. Sprinkle the inside with salt and put the melon in a large deep pan with enough boiling water to cover it. Simmer for 30 minutes, drain, and place it in a large steamer; steam for another 30 minutes. Bring the stock to a boil and pour it into the melon; cover and steam for 25 minutes. Add the ginseng and other ingredients and serve. Add some of the winter-melon flesh, scraped out with a spoon, when ladling the soup into individual bowls. Garnish with cilantro. Makes 6 servings.

Adapted from *The Food of Asia* by Kong Foong Ling, 2002.

CHOCOLATE PEANUT-BUTTER GINSENG COOKIES

1½ cups all-purpose flour

½ cup unsweetened cocoa powder (not Dutch-process)

¾ teaspoon baking soda

¼ teaspoon salt

1 teaspoon powdered ginseng

2 sticks (1 cup) unsalted butter, softened

1 cup granulated sugar

¼ cup packed light-brown sugar

1 large egg

1½ teaspoons vanilla

1⅔ cups (a 10-ounce bag) peanut butter chips

1 cup semisweet chocolate chips (about 8 ounces)

Preheat the oven to 350° F. In a bowl, sift together the flour, cocoa powder, baking soda, salt, and ginseng powder. Beat together the butter and sugars with an electric mixer until light and fluffy; beat in the egg and vanilla until combined well. Beat in the flour mixture until just combined and then stir in the chips.

Drop the dough by tablespoons about 2 inches apart onto an ungreased baking sheet and bake in the middle of the oven until the cookies begin to crack on top (about 12 minutes). Place the cookies on racks to cool. Makes 4–5 dozen cookies.

Adapted from www.epicurious.com and www.hsuginseng.com.

SOURCES

INTRODUCTION

Bodeker, G. C. Introduction, *Medicinal Plants for Forest Conservation and Health Care.* Food and Agricultural Organization of the United Nations, Rome. 1997.

1: THE ROOT AT HAND

Beyfuss, Bob, ed. American Ginseng Production in the 21st Century. Conference Proceedings. Cornell Cooperative Extension of Greene County. September 2000.

Bilger, Burkhard. "Wild 'Sang." *The New Yorker,* July 15, 2002.

Briggs, J. C. *Biogeography and Plate Tectonics.* New York: Elsevier, 1987.

Kauffman, Gary L. "American ginseng *Panax quinquefolius,*" in *Management Indicator Species Habitat and Population Trends, Nantahala and Pisgah National Forest.* Unpublished report by the National Forests in North Carolina, Asheville, NC (division of U.S. Department of Agriculture). 2001.

Messerli, B., and J. D. Ives, ed. *Mountains of the World: A Global Priority.* New York: Parthenon Publishing Group, 1997.

2: THE DOCTORS DEBATE

Beinfield, Harriet, and Efrem Korngold. *Between Heaven and Earth: A Guide to Chinese Medicine.* New York: Ballantine Books, 1992.

Bensky, Dan, and Andrew Gamble, eds. *Chinese Herbal Medicine: Materia Medica.* Seattle: Eastland Press, 1986.

Camporesi, Piero. *Exotic Brew: The Art of Living in the Age of Enlightenment.* Trans. by Christopher Woodall. Cambridge, UK: Polity Press, 1994.

Coleman, C. I., J. H. Hebert, and P. Reddy. "The effects of *Panax ginseng* on quality of life." *Journal of Clinical Pharmacy and Therapeutics* 28 (2003): 5–15.

Ellis, Jennifer M., and Prabashni Reddy. "Effects of *Panax ginseng* on quality of life." *Annals of Pharmacotherapy* 36 (3):375–79. 2002.

Foster, Steven. "Phytogeographic and botanical considerations of medicinal plants in eastern Asia and eastern North America." In *Herbs, Spices, and Medicinal Plants,* vol. 4. Edited by Lyle E. Craker and James E. Simon. Phoenix: Oryx Press, 1989.

Furth, Charlotte. *A Flourishing Yin: Gender in China's Medical History, 960–1665.* Berkeley: University of California Press, 1999.

Gordon, James. *Manifesto for a New Medicine: Your Guide to Healing Partnerships and the Wise Use of Alternative Therapies.* New York: Addison-Wesley, 1996.

Hou, Joseph P. *The Myth and Truth About Ginseng.* South Brunswick, NJ: A.S. Barnes & Co., 1978.

Jarvis, William T., and Stephen Barrett. "How quackery sells." http://www.quackwatch.org/. Adapted from Stephen Barrett and William T. Jarvis, eds. *The Health Robbers: A Closer Look at Quackery in America.* Amherst, NY: Prometheus Books, 1995.

Lewis, Walter H., and P. F. Memory Elvin-Lewis. *Medical Botany: Plants Affecting Human Health,* second edition. New York: John Wiley & Sons, 2003.

Lindley, John. *Natural System of Botany; or, A Systematic View of the Organisation, Natural Affinities, and Geographical Distribution of the Whole Vegetable Kingdom,* second edition. London: Longman, 1836.

Needham, Joseph. *Science and Civilisation in China,* vol. 6, *Biology and Biological Technology.* New York: Cambridge University Press, 1996.

Reston, James. "A View from Shanghai." *The New York Times,* August 22, 1971, E13.

———. *Deadline: A Memoir.* New York: Random House, 1991.

Rosen, Samuel. "I Have Seen the Past, and It Works." *The New York Times,* November 1, 1971, 41.

Shiu Ying Hu. "The Genus *Panax* (ginseng) in Chinese Medicine." *Economic Botany* 30: 11–28. January–March, 1976.

Smithies, Michael, ed. *Aspects of the Embassy to Siam 1685, by the Chevalier de Chaumont and the Abbé de Choisy.* Chiang Mai, Thailand: Silkworm Books, 1997.

Thompson, Gary A. "Botanical Characteristics of Ginseng." In *Herbs, Spices, and Medicinal Plants,* vol. 2. Edited by Lyle E. Craker and James E. Simon. Phoenix. Phoenix: Oryx Press, 1989.

Tyler, Varro. *Tyler's Honest Herbal: A Sensible Guide to the Use of Herbs and Related Remedies,* fourth edition. Edited by Steven Foster and Varro E. Tyler. Binghamton, NY: Haworth Press, 1999.

————. Author interview, June 2001.

Vuksan, V., J. L. Sievenpiper, V. Y. Koo, T. Francis, U. Beljan-Zdravkovic, Z. Xu, and E. Vidgen. "American ginseng (*Panax quinquefolius* L.) reduces postprandial glycemia in nondiabetic subjects and subjects with type 2 diabetes mellitus." *Archives of Internal Medicine* 160 (7) (April 10, 2000):1009–13.

Vuksan, V., J. L. Sievenpiper, J. Wong, Z. Xu, U. Beljan-Zdravkovic, J. T. Arnason, V. Assinewe, M. P. Stavro, A. L. Jenkins, L. A. Leiter, and T. Francis. "American ginseng (*Panax quinquefolius* L.) attenuates postprandial glycemia in a time-dependent but not dose-dependent manner in healthy individuals." *American Journal of Clinical Nutrition* 73 (4) (April 2001): 753–58.

Winter, Greg. "FDA Warns Food Companies about Herbal Additives." *The New York Times,* June 7, 2001, C1.

Xiao Pei-Gen and Fu Shan-Lin. "Pharmacologically Active Substances of Chinese Traditional and Herbal Medicines." In *Herbs, Spices, and Medicinal Plants: Recent Advances in Botany, Horticulture, and Pharmacology,* vol. 2. Edited by Lyle E. Craker and James E. Simon. Phoenix: Oryx Press, 1987.

3: THE EMPEROR'S FAVORITE

"Hidden New York: 32 Mott Street General Store." PBS website. http://www.pbs.org/wnet/newyork/hidden/contents.html.

Dharmananda, Subhuti. "The nature of ginseng: Traditional use, modern research, and the question of dosage." *HerbalGram* 54: 34–51. 2002.

Fairbank, John K., ed. *The Cambridge History of China,* vol. 10. New York: Cambridge University Press, 1978.

Hosie, Alexander. *Manchuria: Its People, Resources and Recent History.* London: Methuen & Co., 1901.

Hummel, Arthur W. *Eminent Chinese of the Ch'ing Period (1644–1912),* vol. 1. U.S. Government Printing Office, Washington, DC. 1943.

Hsu, Immanuel C. Y. *The Rise of Modern China,* sixth edition. New York: Oxford University Press, 2000.

Symons, Van Jay. *Ch'ing Ginseng Management: Ch'ing Monopolies in*

Microcosm. Occasional Paper No. 13, Center for Asian Studies, Arizona State University. March 1981.

4: LIFE IN A NEW WORLD

Thanksgiving Address. Native Self-Sufficiency Center, Six Nations Indian Museum Tracking Project. Corrales, New Mexico. n.d.

Appleby, John H. "Ginseng and the Royal Society." *Notes and Records of the Royal Society of London,* 1983. 37(2): 121–146.

Brunk, Robert S., ed. *May We All Remember Well,* vol. 1. Robert S. Brunk Auction Services, Asheville, N.C. 1997.

Canadian Pacific Railway. "Ginseng in Canada." *Agricultural and Industrial Progress in Canada* 4 (10) (October 1922).

Davis, Donald E. *Where There Are Mountains: An Environmental History of the Southern Appalachians.* Athens, GA: University of Georgia Press, 2000.

Fenton, William Nelson. "Contacts between Iroquois Herbalism and Colonial Medicine." *Annual Report of the Smithsonian Institution.* Washington, DC. 1941.

Fenton, William N., and Elizabeth L. Moore. Introduction, *Customs of the American Indians Compared with the Customs of Primitive Times,* by J. F. Lafitau. Toronto: Champlain Society, 1974.

Foster, Martha Harroun. "Lost women of the matriarchy: Iroquois women in the historical literature." *American Indian Culture and Research Journal* 19(3): 121–40. 1995.

Goldstein, Beth. "Ginseng: Its History, Dispersion, and Folk Tradition." *American Journal of Chinese Medicine* 3 (3): 223–34. 1975.

Herrick, James W. *Iroquois Medical Botany.* Syracuse: Syracuse University Press, 1995.

Horton, James H., Theda Perdue, and James M. Gifford. *Our Mountain Heritage: Essays on the Natural and Cultural History of Western North Carolina.* Raleigh: North Carolina Humanities Committee, 1979.

Lafitau, Joseph-Francois. Memoire presente a son Altesse royale Monseigneur le duc d'Orleans, regent du royaume de France: concernant la precieuse plant du gin-seng de Tartarie, decouverte en Canada par le P. Joseph Francois Lafitau, de la Compagnie de Jesus, Missionaire des Iroquois du Sault Saint Louis. Chez Joseph Monge, Rue St. Jacques, Paris. 1718.

Motsch, Andreas. *Lafitau et l'emergence du discours ethnographique.* Montreal: Septentrion, 2001.

Rossman, Douglas A. *Where Legends Live: A Pictorial Guide to Cherokee Mythic Places.* Cherokee, NC: Cherokee Publications, 1988.

Silver, Timothy. *A New Face on the Countryside: Indians, Colonists, and Slaves in South Atlantic Forests, 1500–1800.* New York: Cambridge University Press, 1990.

Sivertsen, Barbara J. *Turtles, Wolves, and Bears: A Mohawk Family History.* Westminister, MD: Heritage Books, 1996.

Snow, Dean R., Charles T. Gehring, and William A. Starna. *In Mohawk Country: Early Narratives about a Native People.* Syracuse: Syracuse University Press, 1996.

Williams, Samuel Cole, ed. *Adair's History of the American Indians.* New York: Promontory Press, 1974.

5: Pursued by Trappers

Hammon, Neal O., ed. *My Father, Daniel Boone: The Draper Interviews with Nathan Boone.* Lexington: The University Press of Kentucky, 1999.

Hankins, Andy. "China–West Virginia ginseng research interchange." Unpublished report. n.d.

Hufford, Mary. "American ginseng and the idea of the commons." Library of Congress website, http://memory.loc.gov/ammem/cmnshtml/essay1/index.html.

———. "Stalking the mother forest: Voices beneath the canopy." *Folklife Center News* 17 (5) (Summer 1995): 10–18. Washington, DC: Library of Congress.

Paine, Albert Bigelow. *Mark Twain: A Biography,* vol. 1. New York: Harper & Brothers, 1912.

Pollan, Michael. *The Botany of Desire: A Plant's Eye View of the World.* New York: Random House, 2001.

6: Courted by Traders, and Dancing the Ginseng Polka

Christman, Margaret C. S. *Adventurous Pursuits: Americans and the China Trade, 1784–1844.* Washington, DC: Smithsonian Institution Press, 1984.

Lass, William. "Ginseng rush in Minnesota." *Minnesota History* 41 (6) (Summer 1969): 249–66.

Lee, Jean Gordon. *Philadelphians and the China Trade, 1784–1844.* Philadelphia: Philadelphia Museum of Art, 1984.

London, Jack. *The Jacket.* 1914. Republished by New York: Horizon Press, 1969.

Morison, Samuel Eliot. *The Maritime History of Massachusetts, 1783– 1860.* New York: Houghton Mifflin Co., 1921.

———. Ohsman & Sons Co. *Journal of Commerce* Nov. 8, 1991.

Smith, Philip Chadwick Foster. *The Empress of China.* Philadelphia: Philadelphia Maritime Museum, 1984.

Thoreau, Henry D. *Journal,* vol. 3 (September 1856 entries). Edited by John C. Broderick. Princeton, NJ: Princeton University Press, 1981.

7: TRADERS AGAIN

Madsen, Axel. *John Jacob Astor: America's First Multimillionaire.* New York: John Wiley & Sons, 2001.

8: OUTLAWS ON THE ROAD TO NOWHERE

Isbell, Robert. *The Last Chivaree: The Hicks Family of Beech Mountain.* Chapel Hill: University of North Carolina Press, 1996.

Kim So-young. "Man to Pay for Wild Ginseng Mistake." *The Korea Herald,* August 9, 2004.

Robbins, Christopher. "TRAFFIC Explores Eco-labeling as a Conservation Tool for American Ginseng." Unpublished paper prepared by TRAFFIC North America. 2002.

———. "Eco-labels may promote market-driven medicinal plant conservation." *HerbalGram* 56: 34 ff. 2002.

9: TAMED, BUT NOT

Carlson, Alvar W. "Ginseng: America's botanical drug connection to the Orient." *Economic Botany* 40 (2): 233–49. 1986.

Hardacre, Val. *Woodland Nuggets of Gold.* New York: Vantage Press, 1968.

Paja Thao, Xa Thao, and Dwight Conquergood. *I Am a Shaman.* Recorded in Chicago. 1984. *The Hmong World* 1: 164–93.

Peckham, Pat. "Man Hopes Drink Boosts Ginseng Market." *Wausau Daily Herald,* April 18, 2002, 1A.

Persons, W. Scott. *American Ginseng: Green Gold,* revised edition. Asheville, NC: Bright Mountain Books, 1994.

Pinkerton, Kathrene. *Bright with Silver.* New York: William Sloane, 1947.

Williams, L. O. "Ginseng." *Economic Botany* 11: 344–48. 1957.

10: SHANGHAIED ONCE MORE

U.S. Department of Agriculture, Foreign Agricultural Service, http://www.fas.usda.gov/.

Duke, James A. "Phytomedicinal forest harvest in the United States." In *Medicinal Plants for Forest Conservation and Health Care.* Rome: Food and Agricultural Organization of the United Nations, 1997.

11: SERVED BY THE FINEST CHEFS

Nation's Restaurant News 33 (21): 78. May 24, 1999.

People Weekly. "Ming Tsai: Chef." People's 50 Most Beautiful People in the World. May 8, 2000.

Schillinger, Liesl. "Ming's Thing." *The New Yorker,* November 15, 1999: 60–67.

Tan Bee Hong. "Laughing Prawns and Pots of Gold." *New Straits Times,* Food, 7, January 21, 2001.

12: BACK IN CHINA

"Investment guide in Puning city." Website for Jieyang, China. http://www.jieyang.gd.cn/TZZN/localintro_pn-e.html/

Hessler, Peter. *River Town.* New York: HarperCollins, 2001.

Ho, I. S. H., and F. C. Leung. "Isolation and characterization of repetitive DNA sequences from *Panax ginseng.*" *Molecular Genetics and Genomics* 266: 951–61. 2002.

Hong Kong Tatler. "Sexual Healing." *Tatler,* February 2003: 101–105.

Leung, F. C., and I. S. H. Ho. "Development of low-cost DNA probe for fingerprinting Asian and North American ginseng." Paper presented at "INABIS '98: Fifth Internet World Congress on Biomedical Sciences," at McMaster University, Canada, Dec. 7–16, 1998.

APPENDIX

Kong Foong Ling. *The Food of Asia.* Singapore: Periplus Editions (HK) Ltd., 2002.

Loecher, Barbara, et al. *New Choices in Natural Healing for Women:*

Drug-Free Remedies from the World of Alternative Medicine. Emmaus, PA: Rodale Press, 1999.

Persons, W. Scott. *American Ginseng: Green Gold,* revised edition. Asheville, NC: Bright Mountain Books, 1994.

For Information on Wild Ginseng Conservation:

Plant Conservation Alliance, National Park Service: www.nps.gov/plants

United Plant Savers: www.unitedplantsavers.org

American Botanical Council: www.herbalgram.org

INDEX